SCIENCE *of*

REACH YOUR FLEXIBLE POTENTIAL, STAY ACTIVE, MAXIMIZE MOBILITY

STRETCH

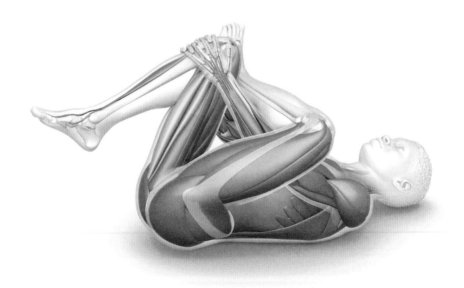

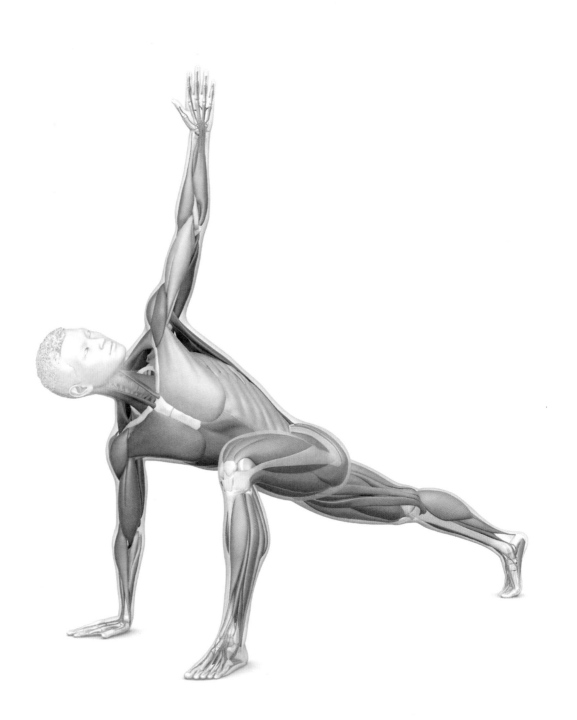

SCIENCE *of*

REACH YOUR FLEXIBLE POTENTIAL, STAY ACTIVE, MAXIMIZE MOBILITY

STRETCH

DR LEADA MALEK, PT, DPT

CONTENTS

PREFACE

Our global society is living in the midst of a physical activity paradox. Despite modern conveniences, we face escalating rates of physical inactivity, yet also a growing initiative advocating for more movement and more understanding of our own bodies.

Physical activity, in its various forms, is the cornerstone of a healthy lifestyle and is a tool to manage and reduce disease risk. It enhances quality of life, instils a sense of purpose, and has the potential to lessen the reliance on medications – notably opioids – for pain management. The effects of exercise on mental and physical health are countless: from helping with symptoms of anxiety, stress, and depression, to improving heart health, bone strength, and longevity.

We often take everyday physical demands and the requisite strength and flexibility to live comfortably for granted, until we lose them, for instance through injury or the aging process. Getting sidelined by pain or simply being overwhelmed by what society paints exercise to look like can be a barrier to progress. A recurring question I receive as a physical therapist is, "What about stretching?"

While the answer often depends on the individual and their goals, this book offers a comprehensive explanation, honouring the intricacies of anatomy and physiology. I find the human body incredibly fascinating, and I believe that a deeper understanding empowers people to cultivate positive beliefs about the body, improve injury outcomes, and ultimately, lead healthier, more active lives.

This book aims to:
1. Introduce anatomy and the science of movement.
2. Reduce barriers to physical activity.
3. Provide a collection of flexibility exercises suitable for various life stages and activities.
4. Promote a healthy lifestyle attuned to the body's adaptability.

The science and discourse surrounding stretching and physical activity have evolved over time and continue to do so with ongoing research. This book seeks to demystify stretching, spotlight a range of techniques to improve flexibility, and consolidate the most recent scientific evidence to assist readers in making informed decisions about their stretching journey.

I want to emphasize the importance of patience, commitment, and above all, kindness towards yourself on this journey. Our bodies are all unique, and progress will look different for everyone. It's crucial to listen to your body, tune into its needs, and celebrate each small victory along the way. In the end, the goal is to foster a deep appreciation for the human body

> # " "
>
> *Flexibility training can positively impact mobility and serve as a gateway to an active lifestyle, fostering an appreciation for the body and its abilities.*

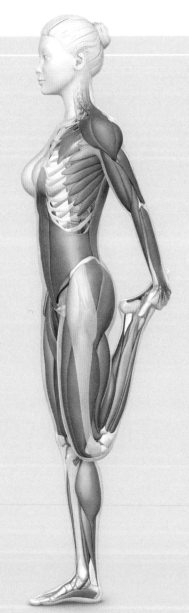

and what it takes to remain active – not just in the short term, but for life.

Writing this book has given me the unique opportunity to educate others about my passion: the human body and movement. It's allowed me to challenge my own biases, in pursuit of the best information. This book is your guide to movement exploration that extends beyond passive static stretching – it is a celebration of the human body and the beautiful, complex ways in which it moves.

I sincerely hope that *Science of Stretch* will serve as a resource on your path towards a more active, healthier lifestyle. May these pages empower and inspire you to prioritize exercise and live a life enriched by meaningful movement, in all its unique forms that resonate with you. I hope you will grow to love it as much as I do!

Leada Malek, PT, DPT, CSCS
Board-Certified Clinical Specialist in Sports
Physical Therapy
Certified Strength and Conditioning Specialist

INTRODUCTION

Stretching has been practised for centuries in ancient civilizations like India, through yoga, and China, through qigong practices. However, it wasn't until the 1940s that stretching became a popular fitness trend and flexibility became highly valued in the West. Our understanding of stretching has evolved greatly.

" "

Try different stretch types, durations, and intensities as you explore movement. Ultimately, the stretch you choose will depend on your movement goals.

ABOUT THIS BOOK

In the world of fitness, understanding the role and impact of stretching can be challenging. Views vary based on personal experience, age, and exposure to information. This book consolidates the latest evidence, so you can make informed decisions about your physical wellness.

We've been taught about stretching since our early schooldays. However, research has revealed that stretching is more nuanced than we initially thought. For example, the type of stretch and how or when it is performed can impact the results on a practitioner. We can also use stretching to improve our day-to-day movement or supporte athletic endeavours.

This book introduces human anatomy, physiology, and even an understanding of the nervous system and pain science to help offer insights into the suitability and benefits of different stretches. It provides a variety of exercises catering to all levels, along with routines to complement your chosen physical activities.

Incorporating stretching into your life requires a commitment. The benefits of flexibility training are significant, but physical wellbeing encompasses not only stretching, but also regular physical activity, a positive mindset, and adequate recovery. Bear in mind the uniqueness of your body, the evolving nature of scientific evidence, and the irreplaceable value of a personalized approach in achieving optimal outcomes.

Use this book as a companion as you embark on your movement journey. You can start at any point – no one is ever too old or too young to begin. Enjoy the process of exploring new facets of physical activity and appreciating the intricate details of your unique body.

A note on terminology

The following definitions will be used in this book: range of motion (ROM) is the degree of movement occurring at a joint. Stretching is a movement applied by an external or internal force in order to increase one's joint ROM. Flexibility refers to the ability of a muscle to lengthen and allow a joint, or joints, to move through a ROM. Mobility refers to the capacity to move efficiently with adequate flexibility, stability, and motor control within a joint or through a movement pattern.

MYTH BUSTING

In this section, we will debunk common myths about stretching, shedding light on misunderstandings and bringing much-needed nuance to this widely discussed yet often misunderstood topic.

MYTH

FACT

> Stretching prevents
> all injuries

STRETCHING ALONE IS NOT SUFFICIENT TO PREVENT ALL-CAUSE INJURIES

Although research supports stretching to help combat the risk of musculotendinous injuries and muscle strains, its ability to prevent all-cause injury is inconclusive. Injury risk reduction training should include an individualized approach (see p.50).

> Stretching eliminates
> muscle soreness

STRETCHING DOES NOT SIGNIFICANTLY AFFECT DELAYED-ONSET MUSCLE SORENESS (DOMS)

Stretching to combat DOMS has only shown very minimal changes in muscle soreness up to 72 hours following exercise.

> All stretching is the same

THERE ARE MANY TYPES OF STRETCHES AND ALL UTILIZE DIFFERENT PARAMETERS

Most people think of the static, passive, type when the word "stretching" is mentioned. However, there are many other types of stretches that are used and different ways they can be classified, including active, dynamic stretches (see p. 40).

> Stretching before exercise can
> negatively impact performance

STATIC STRETCHING MAY NEGATIVELY AFFECT PERFORMANCE, BUT DYNAMIC STRETCHING MAY POSITIVELY AFFECT IT

If a sport requires a significant range of motion (e.g. gymnastics or martial arts), dynamic stretching prior to exercise can improve flexibility and thus enhance performance.

> Stretching only causes changes
> in the nervous system

BOTH NEURAL AND STRUCTURAL CHANGES OCCUR WITH STRETCHING

Besides neural changes when stretching, changes also occur at tissue level. For example, tissue stiffness in muscles and tendons, muscle fascicle length, and even changes in the small blood vessel structures (see p.44) can accompany stretching.

PHYSIOLOGY OF **STRETCHING**

An understanding of human anatomy and physiology is crucial to fully appreciate the mechanics of movement and the importance of physical activity throughout the lifespan. This section explores the highly adaptable human body, the musculoskeletal and nervous systems, the brain, and pain science. Throughout, it spotlights stretching and its benefits at every age.

ANATOMY OF MOVEMENT

Physical activity and exercise require purposeful movement. This entails the body acting on the environment through movements that are a result of muscle contractions organized by the nervous system.

The brain controls voluntary movement. The motor cortex, located just behind the frontal lobe, initiates a signal through the brain and spinal cord. Motor neurons activate the skeletal muscle cells or fibres to contract. Neuromuscular activity is supported by the respiratory and cardiovascular system in the continuous delivery of oxygen to the working tissues. Proprioceptive and sensory feedback allows the body to move in responses to changes in the environment or state of the body.

Limbs
Move towards a target or goal position

Visual system
Detects and interprets light stimuli and works with the vestibular system (see below) as the body moves

Motor cortex
The motor cortex in the brain generates and sends a message to the muscles being commanded

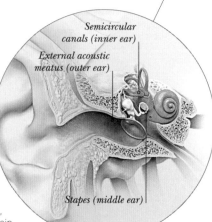

Semicircular canals (inner ear)

External acoustic meatus (outer ear)

Stapes (middle ear)

Vestibular system
The vestibular system is used to maintain equilibrium. The semicircular canals detect head rotation and are sensitive to angular acceleration. The otolith organs detect gravitational forces and are sensitive to linear acceleration. This sensory information is used for balance, to detect head position, and to maintain a stable visual gaze.

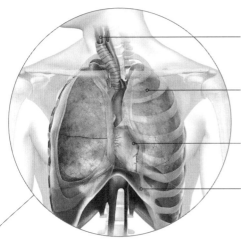

The trachea is the main airway passage

The lungs oxygenate the blood and expel carbon dioxide

The heart pumps blood throughout the body

The diaphragm aids with breathing by contracting

Cardiovascular and respiratory systems

The cardiovascular system delivers blood to the tissues, providing essential nutrients to the cells and removing waste from them. The respiratory system exchanges oxygen (needed for energy) and carbon dioxide (a waste product from energy production) between the environment and the body's cells. This respiratory and circulatory processing increases to meet the body's needs during exercise.

WHAT HAPPENS WHEN WE STRETCH

Stretching begins with movement. The brain coordinates voluntary movement with the muscles to position the body in a way that achieves a tensile, or pulling, force to a target muscle or muscle group. This can be done actively or passively, as demonstrated with various types of stretching. To date, studies have found this yields both neural and non-neural adaptations in skeletal muscle that improve a level of flexibility and joint range of motion. While there is still much to learn, the emerging field of mechanobiology continues to research how cell and tissue mechanics respond to physical forces.

Effects on tissue

Stretching can improve range of motion by increasing fascicle length, improving stretch tolerance, and reducing tonic reflex activity. Some studies have found stretching to improve muscle cross-sectional area and alter pennation angles of muscle fibres.

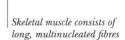

Muscle nuclei

Skeletal muscle consists of long, multinucleated fibres

MOVEMENT IN SPACE
Proprioceptive feedback helps to communicate where the body is in space with the central nervous system. This allows for movement correction, maintenance of postural stability, and spatial awareness.

Strength
Helps maintain muscle tension to sustain joint angles

Extensibility
This is controlled by the contracting muscle

WORLD'S GREATEST STRETCH (SEE P.140)

13

TYPES OF MOTION

The human body functions in several planes of motion. In order to get acquainted with basic movement terminology, it's important to understand the terms used to describe motions and joint positions, and how they relate to the exercises in this book.

The anatomical position (right) is the standard reference orientation of the human body used in science. It allows for a clear and consistent way to describe the locations of structures. The position shows the body standing with feet parallel, toes pointed forward, hands by the side, and palms facing forwards. Three planes of motion pass through the anatomical position and are used to describe movement and orientation.

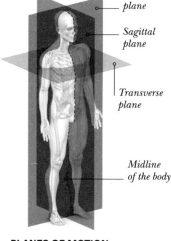

Coronal plane

Sagittal plane

Transverse plane

Midline of the body

PLANES OF MOTION
An exercise can move along one or multiple planes of motion. The coronal and sagittal planes divide the body into front and back, and right and left. Rotational movement occurs along the transverse plane.

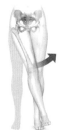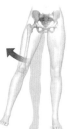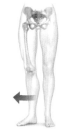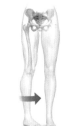

Midline

Right | Left

Medial | Lateral

Lateral

Anterior | Posterior

Superior | Inferior

Proximal | Distal

DESCRIBING LOCATION
Medial and lateral describe something relative to the midline. Front to back is anterior and posterior, respectively. Proximal and distal describe something closer to, or further from an origin.

Spine
The spine helps to transfer load throughout the body. As a whole, it is capable of performing each of these movements.

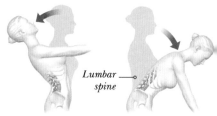

Lumbar spine

EXTENSION
Bending back by extending the spine backwards.

FLEXION
Moving the torso forwards by rounding at the spine.

Elbow
The elbow is the link between the shoulder and hand. It is involved in exercises that require arm and hand use.

EXTENSION
Straightening the arm by moving the forearm down.

FLEXION
Bending the arm by bringing the forearm up.

Hip
This ball-and-socket joint is designed for weightbearing and stability. It is capable of combined and individual motions.

ADDUCTION
Moving the thigh towards the midline.

ABDUCTION
Moving the thigh away from the midline.

EXTERNAL ROTATION
Rotating the thigh outwards.

INTERNAL ROTATION
Rotating the thigh inwards.

ROTATION
Twisting the trunk right or left on the midline.

LATERAL FLEXION
Leaning the trunk right or left from the midline.

Wrist

The wrist flexes, extends, and deviates medially and laterally. Hand supination and pronation occur in the forearm.

SUPINATION
Rotating the forearm to turn palm face up.

PRONATION
Rotating the forearm to turn the palm down.

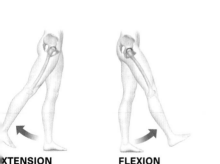

XTENSION
xtending the thigh ackwards, moving the nee behind the hip.

FLEXION
Bringing the thigh forwards, the knee in front of the hip.

Shoulder

The shoulder girdle is made up of the glenohumeral, acromioclavicular, sternoclavicular, and scapulothoracic joints. It is one of the most mobile joints in the body and is capable of a variety of movements.

FLEXION
Moving the arm forwards using the shoulder.

EXTENSION
Moving the arm backwards using the shoulder.

ADDUCTION
Moving the arm towards the midline.

ABDUCTION
Moving the arm away from the midline.

EXTERNAL ROTATION
Rotating the arm outwards at the shoulder.

INTERNAL ROTATION
Rotating the arm inwards at the shoulder.

Knee

The tibiofemoral and patellofemoral joints make up the knee, the largest synovial joint (see p.28) in the body. It is capable of detailed movements, but primarily flexes and extends and is heavily involved in weightbearing.

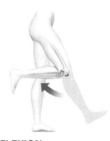

FLEXION
Bending at the knee, bringing the foot closer to the thigh.

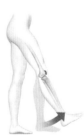

EXTENSION
Straightening at the knee, bringing the foot forward.

Ankle

The ankle is involved in locomotion and articulates with the foot to achieve many motions, including inversion and eversion.

DORSIFLEXION
Pointing the foot and toes upwards.

PLANTARFLEXION
Pointing the foot and toes downwards.

MUSCULAR SYSTEMS

While cardiac and smooth muscle are included in the muscular system, the majority of the body's muscle tissue is skeletal muscle. Skeletal muscle attaches to bones via tendons and pulls on them to create movement.

Muscles are often named because of their shape, position, attachments, or fibre orientation. Skeletal muscle contracts primarily in response to a voluntary stimulus. The four muscle properties that contribute to how it performs under load, like stretching, are: extensibility, elasticity, contractility, and excitability. Individual muscle fibres possess different physiological and structural characteristics that determine their functional capacity.

A zoomed-in view shows myofibrils lined up with one another

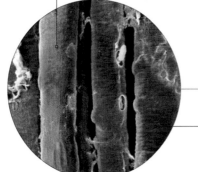

Elbow flexors
Biceps brachii
Brachialis (deep)
Brachioradialis

Visible stripes (striations) reflect the arrangement of muscle proteins

Skeletal muscle fibres
These muscle fibres consist of long, multinucleated, cylindrical cells made up of thousands of myofibrils. They contain proteins that enable muscle contraction.

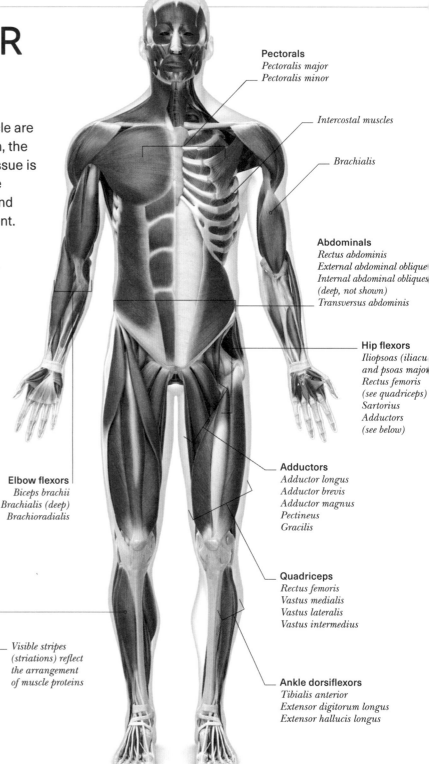

Pectorals
Pectoralis major
Pectoralis minor

Intercostal muscles

Brachialis

Abdominals
Rectus abdominis
External abdominal oblique
Internal abdominal obliques
(deep, not shown)
Transversus abdominis

Hip flexors
Iliopsoas (iliacu
and psoas majo
Rectus femoris
(see quadriceps)
Sartorius
Adductors
(see below)

Adductors
Adductor longus
Adductor brevis
Adductor magnus
Pectineus
Gracilis

Quadriceps
Rectus femoris
Vastus medialis
Vastus lateralis
Vastus intermedius

Ankle dorsiflexors
Tibialis anterior
Extensor digitorum longus
Extensor hallucis longus

SUPERFICIAL   **DEEP**

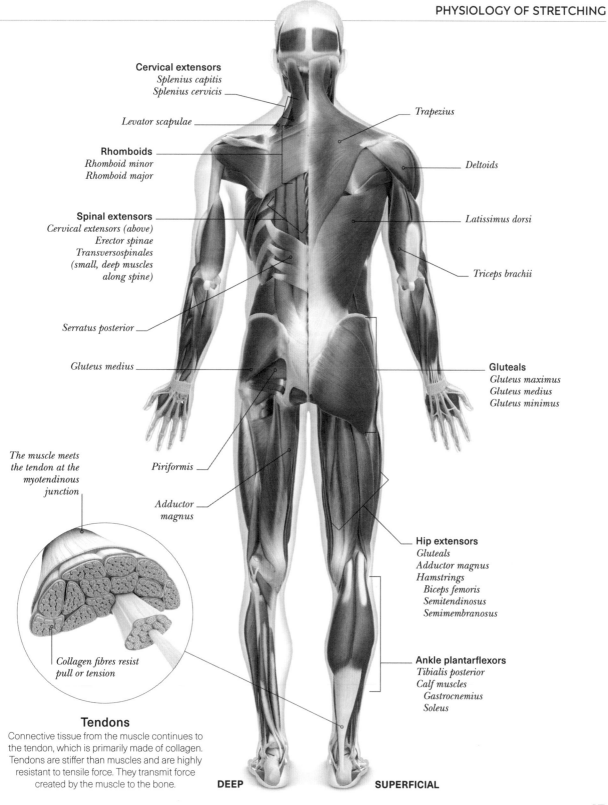

Cervical extensors
Splenius capitis
Splenius cervicis

Levator scapulae

Rhomboids
Rhomboid minor
Rhomboid major

Spinal extensors
Cervical extensors (above)
Erector spinae
Transversospinales
(small, deep muscles
along spine)

Serratus posterior

Gluteus medius

Trapezius

Deltoids

Latissimus dorsi

Triceps brachii

Gluteals
Gluteus maximus
Gluteus medius
Gluteus minimus

*The muscle meets
the tendon at the
myotendinous
junction*

Piriformis

*Adductor
magnus*

*Collagen fibres resist
pull or tension*

Tendons

Connective tissue from the muscle continues to
the tendon, which is primarily made of collagen.
Tendons are stiffer than muscles and are highly
resistant to tensile force. They transmit force
created by the muscle to the bone.

Hip extensors
Gluteals
Adductor magnus
Hamstrings
Biceps femoris
Semitendinosus
Semimembranosus

Ankle plantarflexors
Tibialis posterior
Calf muscles
Gastrocnemius
Soleus

DEEP

SUPERFICIAL

MUSCLE CHAINS AND GROUPINGS

Muscles work as a system to enable the body to move through different planes of motion. Many theories have been proposed to try to categorize muscles and conceptualize how this happens based on biomechanics and anatomy.

Rather than focussing on individual muscle function, it may be helpful to appreciate where muscles are in proximity to the joints they move. The "core" includes global, local, and neighboring muscles and joints from the abdomen, spine, pelvis, and hips. These muscles work together to create and transfer forces through the body.

GLOBAL MUSCLES

Global muscles are more superficial (nearer the surface) than local muscles. They are much larger, and have a greater ability to generate force on the joints they attach to. Global muscles work with the local muscles to help transfer load between the upper and lower extremities. Core training programmes focussing on the global and local muscles individually or together, as well as general exercises, can help with the management of back pain.

Global muscles consist of the quadratus lumborum, psoas major, external and internal obliques, rectus abdominis, gluteus medius, and all of the hip adductor muscles including adductor magnus, longus and brevis, gracilis, and pectineus.

LOCAL MUSCLES

Local muscles are located deep in the body and attach to one or a few vertebrae. Due to their location and proximity to a joint, they naturally have an influence on the control and smaller movements of these

bones. However, they typically cannot create powerful, larger movements. Local core muscles include the diaphragm, multifidi, transversus abdominis, and pelvic floor muscles. Proper coordination of activity between this group can help modulate intra-abdominal pressure, which can affect spinal stiffness, as well as movement, breathing, and continence.

MOVEMENT SYSTEM

Local and global systems work with additional muscles, including the latissimus dorsi, hip flexors, and quadriceps to create movement. There are various theories to help understand how movement is transmitted between muscle groups in the body – like muscle "slings". Since fascia, or connective tissue, exists throughout the body and provides structural support, it can transmit force generated from muscles to the bones. Knowing how muscles work together at or near the trunk can help you choose relevant exercises geared towards your particular movement goals.

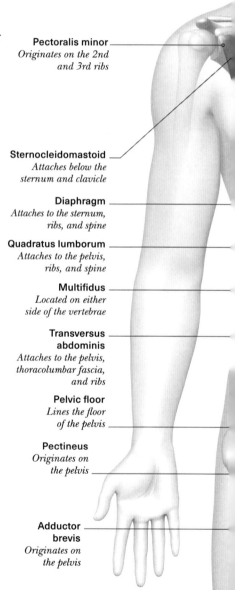

Pectoralis minor
Originates on the 2nd and 3rd ribs

Sternocleidomastoid
Attaches below the sternum and clavicle

Diaphragm
Attaches to the sternum, ribs, and spine

Quadratus lumborum
Attaches to the pelvis, ribs, and spine

Multifidus
Located on either side of the vertebrae

Transversus abdominis
Attaches to the pelvis, thoracolumbar fascia, and ribs

Pelvic floor
Lines the floor of the pelvis

Pectineus
Originates on the pelvis

Adductor brevis
Originates on the pelvis

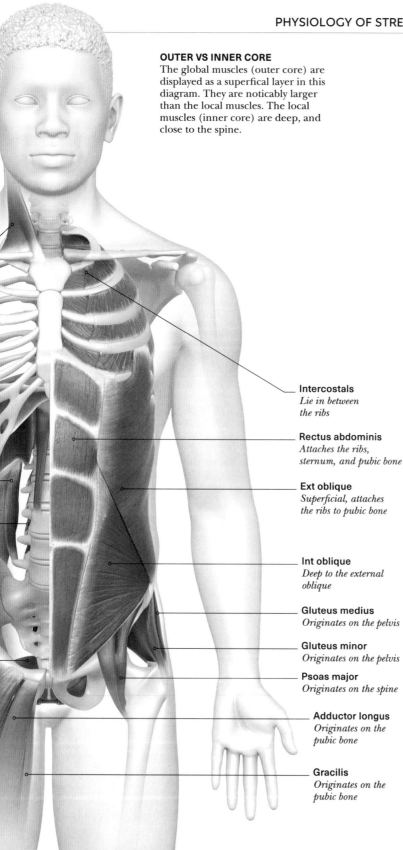

OUTER VS INNER CORE
The global muscles (outer core) are displayed as a superfical layer in this diagram. They are noticably larger than the local muscles. The local muscles (inner core) are deep, and close to the spine.

Intercostals
Lie in between the ribs

Rectus abdominis
Attaches the ribs, sternum, and pubic bone

Ext oblique
Superficial, attaches the ribs to pubic bone

Int oblique
Deep to the external oblique

Gluteus medius
Originates on the pelvis

Gluteus minor
Originates on the pelvis

Psoas major
Originates on the spine

Adductor longus
Originates on the pubic bone

Gracilis
Originates on the pubic bone

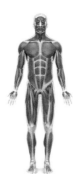

ANTERIOR OBLIQUE SLING
This includes the external obliques, internal obliques, and contralateral adductor muscles. It stabilizes the hip and pelvis and assists with acceleration, rotation, deceleration, and change of direction in sport.

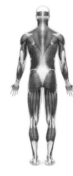

POSTERIOR OBLIQUE SLING
This sling consists of the latissimus dorsi, gluteus maximus, and thoracolumbar fascia. It supports the trunk and pelvis during activities like the stance phase of walking, as well as propulsion (moving forwards).

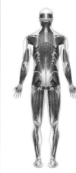

DEEP LONGITUDINAL SLING
This sling includes the erector spinae, multifidus, sacrotuberous ligament, thoracolumbar fascia, and biceps femoris. It assists with forwards and backwards movement and keeping the body upright.

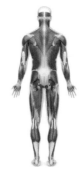

LATERAL SLING
The lateral sling consists of the gluteus medius, gluteus minimus, tensor fascia latae, and illiotibial band. This group helps with frontal plane movement and stabilizes the hip and pelvis during single leg activities.

HOW MUSCLES WORK

Muscles attach to bones via tendons. With voluntary movement, the nervous system generates a signal to the nerves that cause the muscles to contract in a variety of ways. Tendons transmit the force generated by muscles to the bones, enabling joint movement.

Eccentric and concentric contractions are isotonic, which involve a change in muscle length. Isometric contractions involve an active muscle that does not change in length, causing a joint angle to remain the same. Muscle has four properties that affect its performance.

Extensibility refers to a muscle's ability to elongate using an external force. **Elasticity** is its ability to return to its resting length. **Contractility** is the ability to generate active tension, and **excitability** refers to how well a muscle responds to a stimulus.

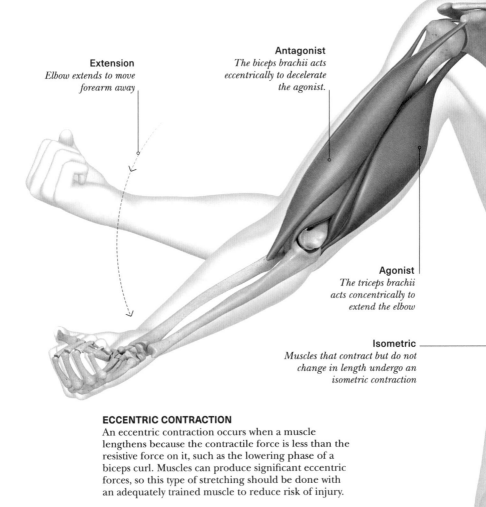

Extension
Elbow extends to move forearm away

Antagonist
The biceps brachii acts eccentrically to decelerate the agonist.

Agonist
The triceps brachii acts concentrically to extend the elbow

Isometric
Muscles that contract but do not change in length undergo an isometric contraction

ECCENTRIC CONTRACTION
An eccentric contraction occurs when a muscle lengthens because the contractile force is less than the resistive force on it, such as the lowering phase of a biceps curl. Muscles can produce significant eccentric forces, so this type of stretching should be done with an adequately trained muscle to reduce risk of injury.

HOW MUSCLES WORK TOGETHER

The muscle primarily causing a movement to occur is an agonist. Those that indirectly assist a movement are synergists. A muscle that can oppose or decelerate the prime mover is the antagonist. Since muscles only pull, they cannot push, these groups all undergo a level of tension for any given movement to occur.

Agonist
The biceps brachii acts concentrically to flex the elbow

CONCENTRIC CONTRACTION
A concentric muscle contraction occurs when a muscle shortens because the contractile force is greater than the resistive force on it, such as in the raising phase of a biceps curl.

Flexion
Bending the elbow to bring the forearm closer

Antagonist
The triceps is the opposing muscle group

Muscle tension

Active tension is the force created when the myosin (thick) and actin (thin) filaments slide past each other within the sarcomeres of a muscle, the force being greatest with a muscle at resting length. Passive tension occurs when a muscle antagonist lengthens with or without an active agonist. As muscle length increases, passive tissues reach their full length and resist further increases in length. Most stretching exercises aim to alter this.

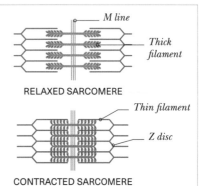

M line

Thick filament

RELAXED SARCOMERE

Thin filament

Z disc

CONTRACTED SARCOMERE

ANATOMY OF A MUSCLE

Skeletal muscle cells are long, cylindrical bundles of smaller fibres called myofibrils. Myofibrils are made up of actin and myosin filaments that slide past each other to create muscle contraction. The cells have mitochondria for energy production and a system of membranes, the sarcoplasmic reticulum, which stores and releases calcium ions to initiate muscle contraction.

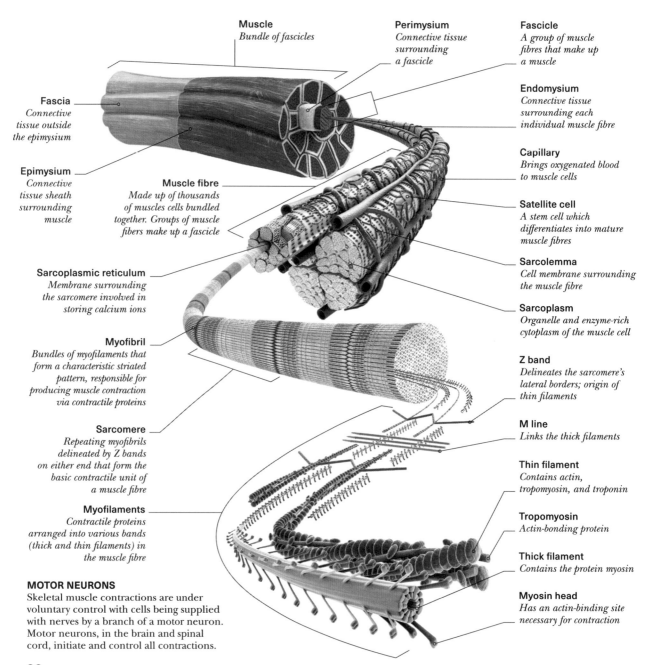

Muscle
Bundle of fascicles

Perimysium
Connective tissue surrounding a fascicle

Fascicle
A group of muscle fibres that make up a muscle

Fascia
Connective tissue outside the epimysium

Endomysium
Connective tissue surrounding each individual muscle fibre

Epimysium
Connective tissue sheath surrounding muscle

Muscle fibre
Made up of thousands of muscles cells bundled together. Groups of muscle fibers make up a fascicle

Capillary
Brings oxygenated blood to muscle cells

Satellite cell
A stem cell which differentiates into mature muscle fibres

Sarcolemma
Cell membrane surrounding the muscle fibre

Sarcoplasmic reticulum
Membrane surrounding the sarcomere involved in storing calcium ions

Sarcoplasm
Organelle and enzyme-rich cytoplasm of the muscle cell

Myofibril
Bundles of myofilaments that form a characteristic striated pattern, responsible for producing muscle contraction via contractile proteins

Z band
Delineates the sarcomere's lateral borders; origin of thin filaments

M line
Links the thick filaments

Sarcomere
Repeating myofibrils delineated by Z bands on either end that form the basic contractile unit of a muscle fibre

Thin filament
Contains actin, tropomyosin, and troponin

Tropomyosin
Actin-bonding protein

Myofilaments
Contractile proteins arranged into various bands (thick and thin filaments) in the muscle fibre

Thick filament
Contains the protein myosin

Myosin head
Has an actin-binding site necessary for contraction

MOTOR NEURONS

Skeletal muscle contractions are under voluntary control with cells being supplied with nerves by a branch of a motor neuron. Motor neurons, in the brain and spinal cord, initiate and control all contractions.

Length-tension relationship

This graph is a basic framework that describes the amount of tension and force a muscle is capable of at different lengths. In general, muscles create greater amounts of tension at shorter lengths and less tension and force at greater lengths as passive tension increases (i.e. end range of a stretch).

KEY
— Total tension
••• Passive tension
▨▨ Active tension

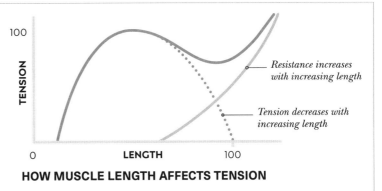

HOW MUSCLE LENGTH AFFECTS TENSION

Resistance increases with increasing length

Tension decreases with increasing length

Muscle contraction at the microscopic level

The shortening and lengthening contractions of skeletal muscle is a complex process that involves the interaction of various proteins and chemical signals. A single motor neuron, and the muscle fibres it supplies with nerves, is a motor unit. Nerve impulses are sent from the motor neuron to muscle fibre, causing the actin filaments to be repeatedly be pulled towards the center of the sarcomere to create tension.

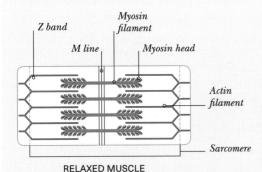

RELAXED MUSCLE

Cross bridges pull the actin filaments to produce tension and contract the muscle.

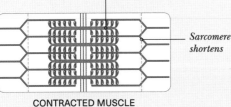

CONTRACTED MUSCLE

Sarcomere shortens

THE CROSS BRIDGE CYCLE

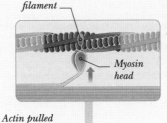

Actin filament

Myosin head

BINDING
The energized myosin head binds to actin, forming a "cross bridge" between the filaments.

Actin pulled along

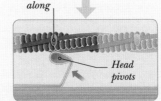

Head pivots

POWER STROKE
ADP and phosphate are released. The myosin head pivots and bends, pulling on the actin filament, sliding it toward the M line.

Cross bridge detaches

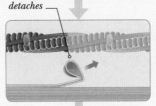

DETACHMENT
An ATP molecule (chemical energy) attaches to myosin, weakening the link between actin and myosin and causing the myosin head to detach.

Myosin re-energized

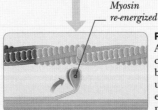

RE-ENERGIZING
ATP releases energy. This causes the myosin head to become reoriented to its upright position and energized, in position for the next cycle.

23

SKELETAL SYSTEM

The adult human skeleton consists of cartilage and bone. It gives the body support, protects vital organs, and allows for movement. Bones are highly specialized, living connective tissue.

Bones continuously renew through our lifespan, as they have the ability to remodel based on the strain placed on them. They serve as reservoirs for essential minerals and bone marrow, which is responsible for the vital task of red blood cell formation. They vary in size, shape, and strength throughout the body.

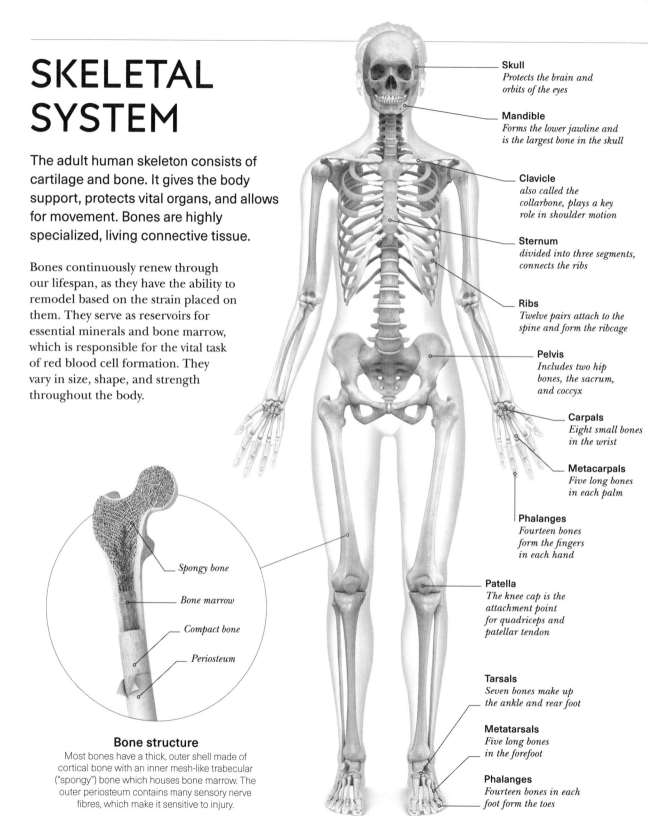

Skull
Protects the brain and orbits of the eyes

Mandible
Forms the lower jawline and is the largest bone in the skull

Clavicle
also called the collarbone, plays a key role in shoulder motion

Sternum
divided into three segments, connects the ribs

Ribs
Twelve pairs attach to the spine and form the ribcage

Pelvis
Includes two hip bones, the sacrum, and coccyx

Carpals
Eight small bones in the wrist

Metacarpals
Five long bones in each palm

Phalanges
Fourteen bones form the fingers in each hand

Patella
The knee cap is the attachment point for quadriceps and patellar tendon

Tarsals
Seven bones make up the ankle and rear foot

Metatarsals
Five long bones in the forefoot

Phalanges
Fourteen bones in each foot form the toes

Spongy bone

Bone marrow

Compact bone

Periosteum

Bone structure
Most bones have a thick, outer shell made of cortical bone with an inner mesh-like trabecular ("spongy") bone which houses bone marrow. The outer periosteum contains many sensory nerve fibres, which make it sensitive to injury.

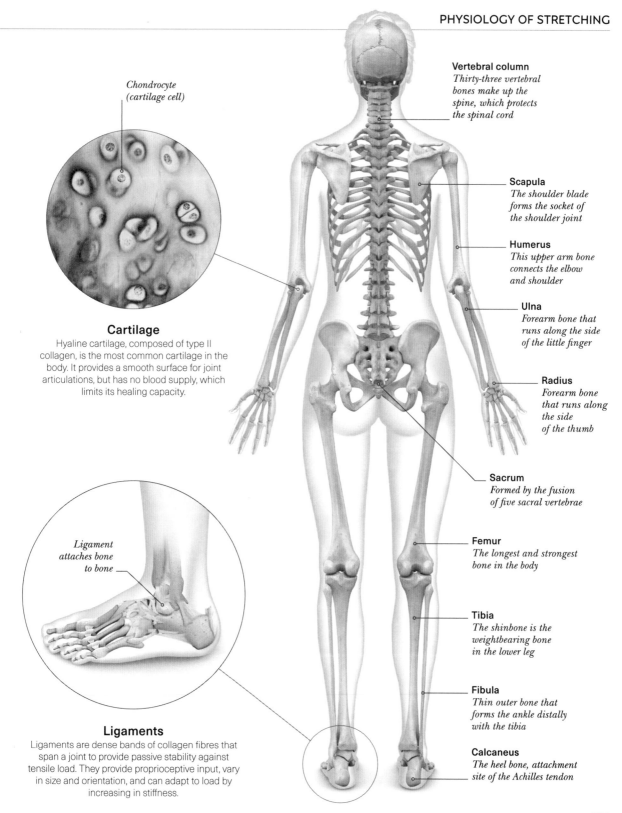

*Chondrocyte
(cartilage cell)*

Cartilage

Hyaline cartilage, composed of type II collagen, is the most common cartilage in the body. It provides a smooth surface for joint articulations, but has no blood supply, which limits its healing capacity.

Ligament attaches bone to bone

Ligaments

Ligaments are dense bands of collagen fibres that span a joint to provide passive stability against tensile load. They provide proprioceptive input, vary in size and orientation, and can adapt to load by increasing in stiffness.

Vertebral column
Thirty-three vertebral bones make up the spine, which protects the spinal cord

Scapula
The shoulder blade forms the socket of the shoulder joint

Humerus
This upper arm bone connects the elbow and shoulder

Ulna
Forearm bone that runs along the side of the little finger

Radius
Forearm bone that runs along the side of the thumb

Sacrum
Formed by the fusion of five sacral vertebrae

Femur
The longest and strongest bone in the body

Tibia
The shinbone is the weightbearing bone in the lower leg

Fibula
Thin outer bone that forms the ankle distally with the tibia

Calcaneus
The heel bone, attachment site of the Achilles tendon

THE SPINE

Typically, the spine is formed of 33 stacked vertebrae. The size of the vertebral bodies increases as it descends to match the weight supported. Natural curves in the spine, both inwards and outwards, exist to allow mechanical balance of the head and body in the sagittal plane. Abnormal curvatures may be congenital or caused by external factors.

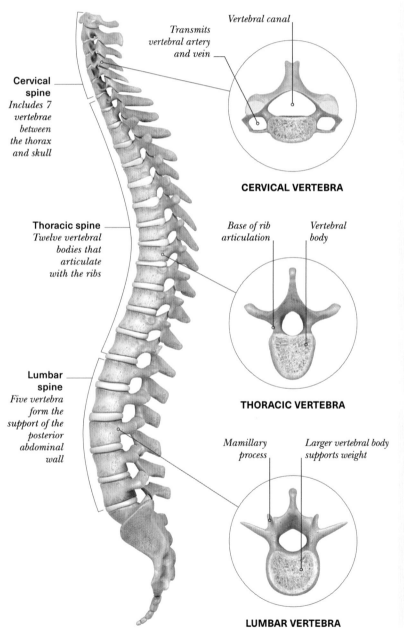

Cervical spine
Includes 7 vertebrae between the thorax and skull

Transmits vertebral artery and vein

Vertebral canal

CERVICAL VERTEBRA

Thoracic spine
Twelve vertebral bodies that articulate with the ribs

Base of rib articulation

Vertebral body

THORACIC VERTEBRA

Lumbar spine
Five vertebra form the support of the posterior abdominal wall

Mamillary process

Larger vertebral body supports weight

LUMBAR VERTEBRA

Posture vs anatomy

Posture is an adaptive response influenced by many things including gravity, mood, movement habits, and anatomy. When it comes to back and neck pain, there is no single "ideal" posture for everyone. Your ideal, or neutral, posture is the position of least resistance for your individual body. Below are some common curvatures.

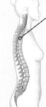

Relaxed, upright posture

NEUTRAL SPINE
Considered to be an efficient position where the head, spine, and pelvis are nearly in line. It is a posture found with the least amount of resistance per individual.

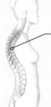

Increased curvature in the thoracic spine

THORACIC KYPHOSIS
Increased curvature in the thoracic spine of greater than 50 degrees. This increased curvature is common with osteoporosis.

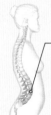

Increased curvature in the lumbar spine

LUMBAR LORDOSIS
Increased lordosis may be present with swayback posture or during pregnancy due to the body's change in centre of mass.

THE PELVIS

The pelvis includes two pelvic bones, the sacrum, and the coccyx. It serves as the connection of the axial skeleton to the lower body and an attachment site for powerful muscles that control the hip and core. The pelvic cavity is continuous with the abdominal cavity and supported by the pelvic floor.

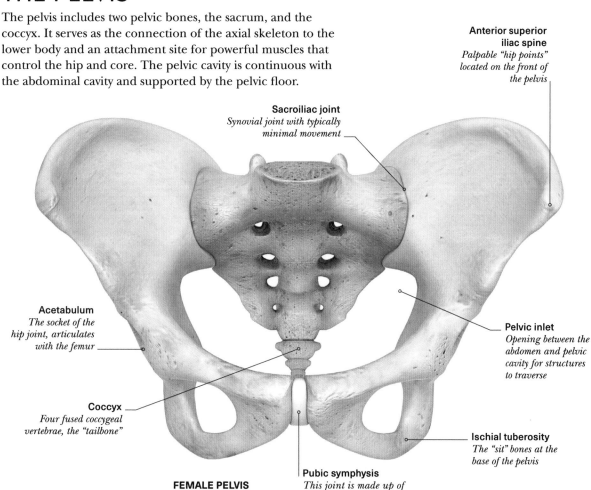

Anterior superior iliac spine
Palpable "hip points" located on the front of the pelvis

Sacroiliac joint
Synovial joint with typically minimal movement

Acetabulum
The socket of the hip joint, articulates with the femur

Pelvic inlet
Opening between the abdomen and pelvic cavity for structures to traverse

Coccyx
Four fused coccygeal vertebrae, the "tailbone"

Ischial tuberosity
The "sit" bones at the base of the pelvis

FEMALE PELVIS

Pubic symphysis
This joint is made up of fibrocartilage, like the discs between vertebrae

Lumbopelvic awareness

Muscle tone, pain, and bone morphology can influence the position of the pelvis and the way it is tilted. Although a neutral pelvis is the ideal position, pelvic tilt can be highly variable among individuals. Understanding lumbopelvic movement may help with controlling core and pelvic position when performing specific exercises.

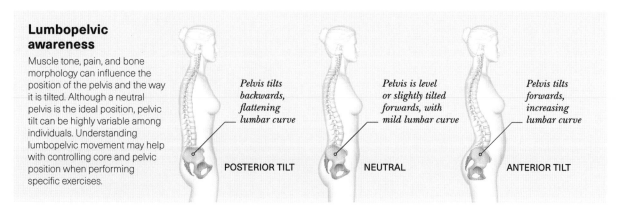

Pelvis tilts backwards, flattening lumbar curve

POSTERIOR TILT

Pelvis is level or slightly tilted forwards, with mild lumbar curve

NEUTRAL

Pelvis tilts forwards, increasing lumbar curve

ANTERIOR TILT

JOINTS

A joint is where two bones make contact. There are three kinds of joints in the body: fibrous, cartilaginous, and synovial. Fibrous joints are fixed, like sutures in the skull. Cartilaginous joints involve cartilage, such as the pubic symphysis.

Synovial joints are the freely mobile, main functional joints in the body. They include hinge joints such as the elbow and knee, that mostly flex and extend. Ball and socket joints, such as the hip and shoulder, have the ability to abduct, adduct, and rotate.

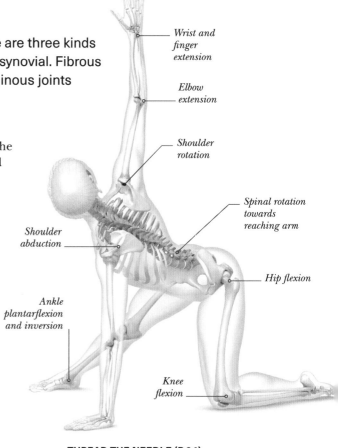

- Wrist and finger extension
- Elbow extension
- Shoulder rotation
- Spinal rotation towards reaching arm
- Shoulder abduction
- Hip flexion
- Ankle plantarflexion and inversion
- Knee flexion

THREAD THE NEEDLE (P.94)

TYPES OF MOVEMENT

Flexion	Joint angle generally gets smaller
Extension	Joint angle generally gets larger
Abduction	Limb moves away from midline or body
Adduction	Limb moves towards midline or body
External rotation	Limb rotates away from body
Internal rotation	Limb rotates inwards towards body
Axial rotation	Spine rotates on its axis
Plantarflexion	Foot points away from body
Dorsiflexion	Foot flexes up towards body

Inside a joint

Synovial joints are characterized by the presence of a joint cavity and by mobility. The synovial membrane, a specialized connective tissue, produces synovial fluid which lubricates and provides nutrients to the articulating surfaces. Fat pads, which occur in the synovial membrane and capsule, can move freely in and out of regions as joints change with movement, serving as a cushion between bones.

SYNOVIAL JOINT

Articular cartilage, a specialized type of connective tissue, covers the articulating surfaces of each bone in the joint. The cartilage provides structural support, cushioning, and gliding.

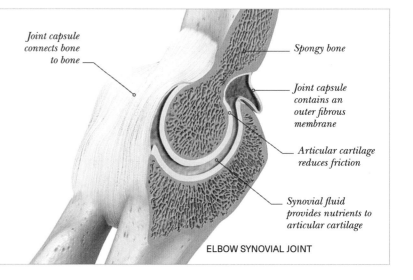

- Joint capsule connects bone to bone
- Spongy bone
- Joint capsule contains an outer fibrous membrane
- Articular cartilage reduces friction
- Synovial fluid provides nutrients to articular cartilage

ELBOW SYNOVIAL JOINT

RANGE OF MOTION

How far a joint can move depends on many factors including muscle, bone structure, soft tissue, ligaments, and bones around it, such as the thigh and calf meeting with knee flexion.

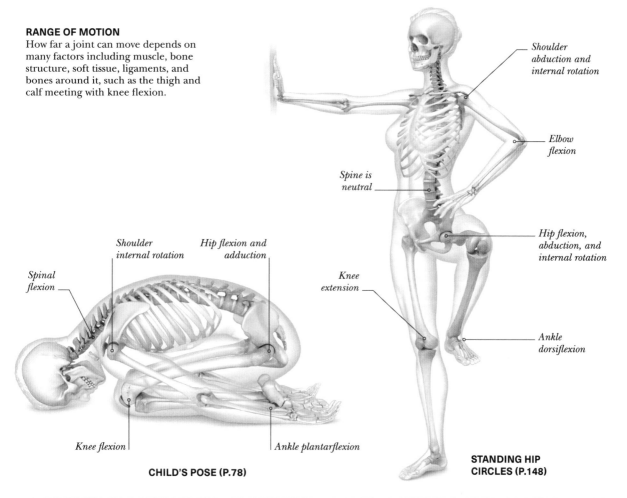

Shoulder abduction and internal rotation

Elbow flexion

Spine is neutral

Hip flexion, abduction, and internal rotation

Knee extension

Ankle dorsiflexion

Spinal flexion

Shoulder internal rotation

Hip flexion and adduction

Knee flexion

Ankle plantarflexion

CHILD'S POSE (P.78)

STANDING HIP CIRCLES (P.148)

Arthritis

Osteoarthritis (OA) is an inflammatory condition where the integrity of the joint tissue undergoes changes. While sometimes asymptomatic, those with early OA symptoms may experience pain and joint stiffness. The main pathological changes of OA include abnormalities in the articular cartilage, synovium, and subchondral bone. Stretching can maintain range of motion and help manage OA.

PROGRESSION

As OA progress, bone swelling, capsular thickening, synovial effusion, and osteophytes (bone spurs) can form, affecting range of motion and joint function.

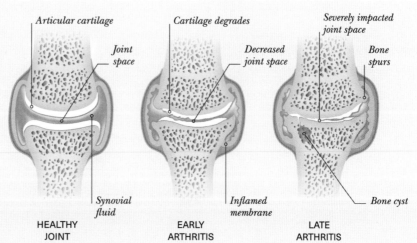

Articular cartilage

Joint space

Cartilage degrades

Decreased joint space

Severely impacted joint space

Bone spurs

Synovial fluid

Inflamed membrane

Bone cyst

HEALTHY JOINT

EARLY ARTHRITIS

LATE ARTHRITIS

NERVOUS SYSTEM

The nervous system is a network of cells, tissues, and organs that control and coordinate the body's responses to internal and external stimuli. It is divided into the central (CNS) and peripheral (PNS) nervous systems.

The CNS includes the brain and spinal cord. It processes and interprets data from the PNS and generates a response. The PNS is divided into the somatic system, which controls voluntary movement and sensory perception, and the autonomic nervous system (ANS), which regulates involuntary functions such as heart rate and breathing. The ANS then further divides into the sympathetic and parasympathetic nervous systems. The nervous system receives sensory information about the body, such as limb position in a stretch, and uses this to adjust and refine movements.

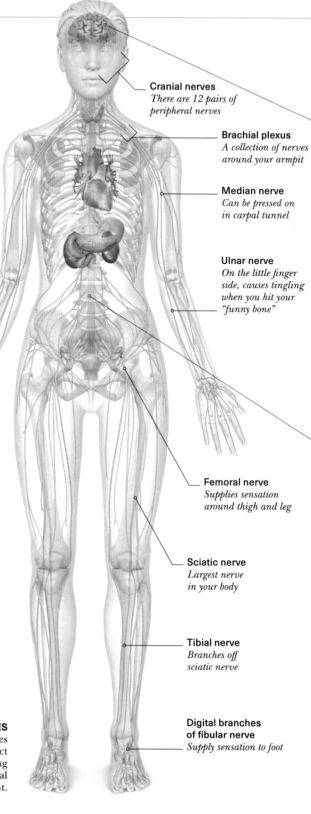

Cranial nerves
There are 12 pairs of peripheral nerves

Brachial plexus
A collection of nerves around your armpit

Median nerve
Can be pressed on in carpal tunnel

Ulnar nerve
On the little finger side, causes tingling when you hit your "funny bone"

Femoral nerve
Supplies sensation around thigh and leg

Sciatic nerve
Largest nerve in your body

Tibial nerve
Branches off sciatic nerve

Digital branches of fibular nerve
Supply sensation to foot

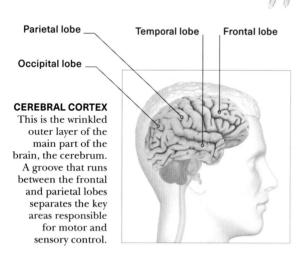

Parietal lobe · Temporal lobe · Frontal lobe

Occipital lobe

CEREBRAL CORTEX
This is the wrinkled outer layer of the main part of the brain, the cerebrum. A groove that runs between the frontal and parietal lobes separates the key areas responsible for motor and sensory control.

PERIPHERAL NERVES
These sensory, motor, and autonomic nerves outside of the brain and spinal cord connect to the rest of the body. By transmitting information between the body and the central nervous system, they control movement.

Pineal gland
Helps regulate sleep-wake cycle

Hypothalamus
Controls body temperature

Cerebellum
Coordinates and controls movement and balance

Pituitary gland
Controls other glands in the body

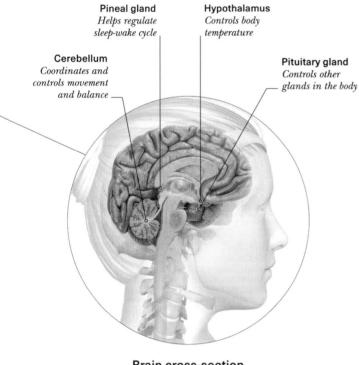

Brain cross-section

The cerebellum helps with motor learning and the planning and execution of smooth, coordinated movements. Important glands in the brain control various body functions by secreting hormones into the bloodstream. Hormones carry messages to organs, muscles, and other tissues.

Spinal cord
Relays body-brain communication signals

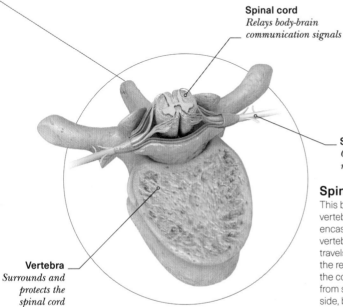

Spinal nerve
Controls sensation and movement of body parts

Spinal cord

This bird's-eye view of a vertebra shows the spinal cord encased within the bony vertebral column. Information travels between the brain and the rest of the body through the cord. Spinal nerves project from small openings on either side, between the vertebrae.

Vertebra
Surrounds and protects the spinal cord

NEURODYNAMICS

Nerves course through the body and must be able to adapt to various loads with movement. The musculoskeletal system serves as the "interface" in which nerves are contained. This includes fascia, skin, bone, muscle, and even blood vessels. In cases of injury or lack of movement, nerves don't undergo their normal stress and may present painful symptoms. Neurodynamic techniques to mobilize them may reduce nerve-related pain.

Biceps

Ulnar nerve

Triceps

Humerus

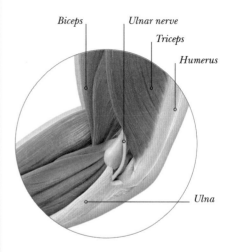

Ulna

MUSCULOSKELETAL INTERFACE
Nerves, which go through muscles and around bones, can be subject to forces like elongation, compression, and gliding. Healthy movement of neural tissue through its mechanical interface, as shown above in a healthy arm, promotes easy movement in the body and limbs.

NATURE AND THEORIES OF PAIN

Everyone experiences pain differently, depending on biological, psychological, and social factors. Understanding the nervous system's role in pain is important for developing effective pain management strategies.

WHAT IS PAIN?

The International Association for the Study of Pain (IASP) defines pain as an "unpleasant sensory and emotional experience associated with, or resembling that associated with, actual or potential tissue damage". Pain can warn the body when it's in danger, such as when touching a hot stove, or when something is wrong, like a broken bone.

Pain can vary widely in intensity, quality, and duration per person. It does not always indicate tissue damage, nor does the intensity always match the level of potential threat. For example, a small paper cut may feel quite painful but likely does not merit surgical intervention.

The IASP notes that pain is "always a personal experience that is influenced to varying degrees by biological, psychological, and social factors," not just sensory neurons. It can be a temporary sensation, caused by a specific injury and subside once the underlying cause is resolved. It can also be chronic, persisting for weeks or years, and have a significant impact on a person's quality of life.

Pain is multifactorial. This offers various options for pain management, including medications or other interventions, like physical therapy. Stretching and exercise can diminish the perception of pain and impact mental wellbeing positively by elevating mood and reducing stress and depression, which are frequently linked to chronic pain conditions. Movement can be an important part of pain management, but consult a healthcare professional to determine what types of exercises are best for individual needs.

CENTRAL SENSITIZATION

The central and peripheral nervous systems are involved in all pain perception pathways. The former interprets information sent from the latter before creating a response or pain signal. Sometimes the brain amplifies this signal, which makes the nervous system hypersensitive to pain and leads to central sensitization. This type of pain can present in various ways including stress, chronic muscoloskeletal pain, stomach pain, or headaches.

What happens with pain?

Many inputs affect how the brain can perceive a threat to the body and its tissues. These play a role in the response, which can manifest as things like muscle pain or anxiety.

- **Sensory input from body**
- **Previous experience**
- **Cultural factors**
- **Social/work environment**
- **Expectations about consequences of threat/danger**
- **Personal beliefs, knowledge, and logic**

ANXIETY EXPECTATION

MEANING/VALUE ATTACHED TO EXPERIENCE

BRAIN RECEIVES LEVEL OF THREAT/DANGER

Outputs are executed to protect the body via pain, motor, immune, nervous system, and endocrine (hormonal) responses.

TYPES OF PAIN

Chronic musculoskeletal pain, such as lower back pain, is the main contributor to disability in the world. According to the World Health Organization, up to 33 per cent of the world's population has some form of musculoskeletal pain. Understanding common types of pain can help with pain management, improving outcomes, and reducing the economic burden.

THREE TYPES OF PAIN

Even though there are many different types of pain, it can be broadly classified into three main types: nociceptive pain, neuropathic pain, and nociplastic pain.

Nociceptive pain arises from actual or threatened damage to non-neural tissue. This pain is usually described as a "sharp" pain and can be localized to a specific site with a clear underlying cause, such as injury or inflammation. Neuropathic pain refers to pain caused by nerve impairment or damage. This pain is usually described by the sufferer as "burning," "shooting," or "throbbing".

Neuropathic pain also manifests with sensory deficits, such as decreased sensation. Complaints of "pins and needles," weakness, or numbness, particularly in the hands and feet, may also present, notably in individuals who are undergoing cancer treatment. Neuropathic pain may also occur with orthopedic conditions (causing a "pinched nerve") or metabolic conditions such as diabetes.

Nociplastic, or psychosomatic, pain may arise from altered nociception despite no clear evidence of tissue damage or threat. The sufferer may feel this pain in several parts of the body at once. It is thought to play a role in chronic pain conditions like lower back pain and fibromyalgia – widespread musculosketal pain that is accompanied by fatigue and memory and mood issues.

REFERRED PAIN

Referred pain is a type of pain felt in a location other than where it originates. The exact mechanisms behind referred pain are not fully understood, but it is thought to be related to the way that the nerves that transmit pain signals are organized in the spinal cord and brain. The nerve pathways that transmit pain signals from different parts of the body converge on the same nerve cells in the spinal cord, and this can cause the brain to be confused when it interprets the signal. For example, the heart may refer pain to the arm, and the liver refer pain to the shoulder. A subcategory of referred pain is radiating pain, when symptoms are felt along the area supplied by a spinal nerve root (see dermatomes diagrams, left).

Referred pain can occur in different patterns, depending on its source, and can help diagnose some medical conditions.

Dermatomes

These are areas of the skin – like a map – that rely on specific nerve connections on the spine. The body has 30 dermatomes: 8 cervical nerves, 12 thoracic nerves, 5 lumbar nerves, and 5 sacral nerves. Each spinal nerve root relays sensory information, such as pain, to the brain from an area on the skin. Dysfunction or damage to a spinal nerve can cause pain in a corresponding zone (see referred pain, right).

KEY

● Trigeminal nerve distribution (provides sensory innervation to the skin of the face)

● Cervical region

● Thoracic region

● Lumbar region

● Sacral region

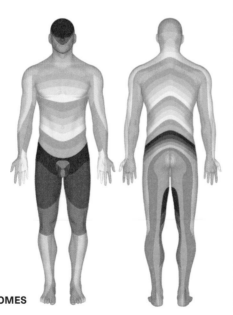

MAP OF DERMATOMES

MOVEMENT AND BRAIN GAINS

The process of moving begins in the brain. The premotor cortex generates a plan, then the primary motor cortex executes it by communicating with the muscles. It does this by sending nerve signals through the main motor pathway that facilitates voluntary movement.

MUSCLE CONTROL

The corticospinal tract is the spinal pathway that is responsible for voluntary movement and communication with muscles. In order to perform a movement, the brain creates a motor plan. Then the brain sends a signal down the corticospinal tract through the spinal cord and to the specific muscle fibres, which contract to move the body as a result.

Other areas of the brain besides the motor cortex are in play when controlling and refining movement. For example, the cerebellum and basal ganglia are involved in coordinating movements and ensuring they are executed smoothly and accurately.

Sensory information from the body, such as awareness of body position and touch, is used to adjust and refine movements as they are being executed.

Overall, movement involves a complex interplay between the brain and multiple regions and systems, all working together to coordinate and execute bodily movements with precision and accuracy.

MOTOR LEARNING
With practice, the nervous system becomes more efficient at controlling movement and reducing unnecessary muscle coactivation because it learns to activate only the necessary muscles for a movement and suppress the unnecessary ones.

Brain
The motor cortex signals the muscles to move, and the sensory cortex receives information from muscles

Spinal cord
Communicates messages to and from the brain

As skill develops, movements become more controlled between the agonist (prime mover) and the antagonist (muscle opposing the prime mover)

SENSORY FEEDBACK TO THE MOTOR CORTEX

SENSORY FEEDBACK TO SPINAL CORD

AGONIST ACTIVATION

ANTAGONIST ACTIVATION

Agonist muscles
The gastrocnemius eccentrically lowers the heels

Antagonist muscles
The ankle dorsiflexors work opposite the plantarflexors

BRAIN HEALTH

Regular exercise has been shown to have neuroprotective effects on the brain by encouraging neurogenesis and neuroplasticity. Increasing blood flow to the brain allows the delivery of oxygen and nutrients to support neurogenesis. Low-intensity exercise, such as walking or stretching, has been shown to increase the production of neurotrophic factors which promote the growth and survival of nerve cells.

Neurogenesis

Exercise can promote the growth of new neurons (nerve cells) in the hippocampus, a brain region that plays a key role in learning and memory. The effects of exercise on this process, called neurogenesis, can benefit people of all ages, including those with neurological disorders such as Alzheimer's disease. Even small amounts of daily activity may have significant benefits for brain health during all stages of life.

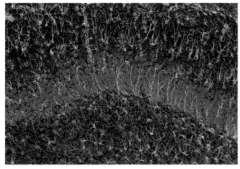

NEW BRAIN CELLS
Neuron cell bodies are coloured pink in this microscopic image of the brain's hippocampus. Exercise promotes the formation of new neurons.

Mind–muscle connection

This refers to the ability to focus on the contraction of specific muscles and visualize the desired movement during exercise. It can enhance muscle activation and promote skill development. By consciously engaging with the targeted muscle group, individuals can improve their motor control and increase their ability to recruit muscle fibres during exercise. This can contribute to muscle growth and strength gains. The mind-muscle connection is often used in resistance training, but can be applied to stretching and other types of exercise as well.

Neuroplasticity

Neuroplasticity is a process that involves adaptive structural and functional changes to the brain. Exercise and physical activity stimulate the brain to form new connections and reorganize existing ones. Movements that are challenging or require learning promote neuroplasticity, as they prompt the brain to adapt and reorganize in response to new demands.

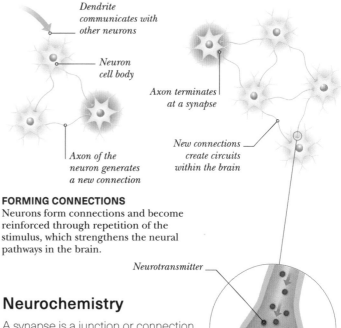

Dendrite communicates with other neurons

Neuron cell body

Axon terminates at a synapse

Axon of the neuron generates a new connection

New connections create circuits within the brain

FORMING CONNECTIONS
Neurons form connections and become reinforced through repetition of the stimulus, which strengthens the neural pathways in the brain.

Neurotransmitter

Neurochemistry

A synapse is a junction or connection point between two neurons where they communicate with each other via neurotransmitters such as dopamine. This communication process between neurons through synapses is how the brain processes and transmits information, and it plays a crucial role in various brain functions such as learning, memory, and movement.

Close-up of synapse
One neuron sends a signal, or neurotransmitter, across the synapse to the other neuron, which then receives the signal and responds accordingly.

RANGE OF MOTION AND FLEXIBILITY

The biomechanics of joint movement, muscle activation, and tissue elasticity all play a role in flexibility, which is typically determined by the range of motion (ROM) around a joint and how the surrounding soft tissues accommodate it.

WHAT HAPPENS WITH A STRETCH?

Put simply, muscles and soft tissues are elongated beyond their resting length, which can lead to various physiological responses in your body during a stretch. The level at which this occurs will depend on individual factors about the person, like age and physiology, and on the stretch parameters utilized, such as intensity and duration.

Someone's ability to move depends on the amount of range of motion available in joints, strength, coordination, and proprioception – the body's ability to sense movement. Since most stretch and mobility training is geared towards improving ROM, it's important to be specific about terms to understand the complexities of the body.

"Joint flexibility" is the available ROM at a joint or series of joints, for example, ankle dorsiflexion requires motion at many joints. ROM can be achieved actively or passively, depending on the tension in the muscles. Someone's active range of motion may be different from their passive range of motion. "Joint mobility" refers to the motion within the joint capsule between articular surfaces. Joint mobility limitations may include changes in joint surfaces, such as with osteoarthritis, as well as the capsule surrounding the joint. "Muscle extensibility" is the muscle's ability to lengthen or elongate with an external force, like contracting the opposing muscle group. "Contractility" is the muscle's ability to forcefully generate tension by pulling on its attachment points. "Elasticity" refers to the muscle returning to its original length after contracting or extending.

REFLEXES

Many events occur in the body to allow you to move into positions to achieve a stretch. Reflexes – mainly the stretch reflex and golgi tendon reflex – protect the body from injury.

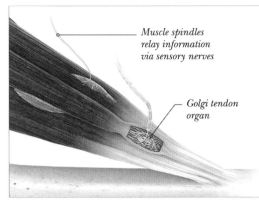

Muscle spindles relay information via sensory nerves

Golgi tendon organ

Feedback to the brain

Muscle spindles are sensory organs within skeletal muscle fibres that detect changes in muscle length. The fibres inside the muscle spindle have sensory nerve endings that trigger a stretch reflex, which causes the muscle to contract to resist further stretching. The golgi tendon organ (GTO) is a sensory receptor located in the tendon of a muscle. The GTO plays an important role in monitoring muscle tension or force during muscle contraction. These two sensory organs work together to regulate muscle length and tension and ensure proper muscle function.

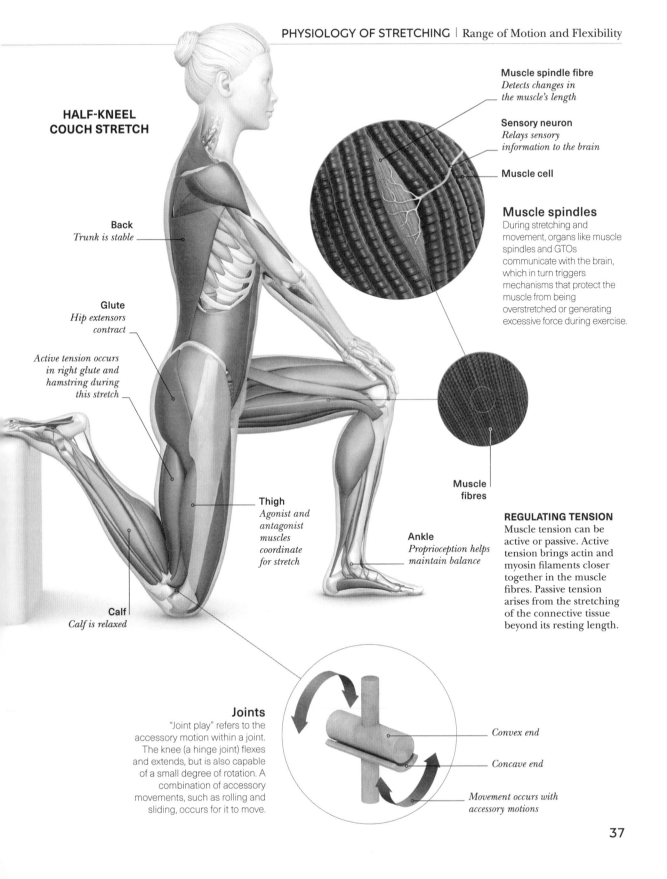

HALF-KNEEL COUCH STRETCH

Muscle spindle fibre
Detects changes in the muscle's length

Sensory neuron
Relays sensory information to the brain

Muscle cell

Muscle spindles
During stretching and movement, organs like muscle spindles and GTOs communicate with the brain, which in turn triggers mechanisms that protect the muscle from being overstretched or generating excessive force during exercise.

Back
Trunk is stable

Glute
Hip extensors contract

Active tension occurs in right glute and hamstring during this stretch

Thigh
Agonist and antagonist muscles coordinate for stretch

Ankle
Proprioception helps maintain balance

Calf
Calf is relaxed

Muscle fibres

REGULATING TENSION
Muscle tension can be active or passive. Active tension brings actin and myosin filaments closer together in the muscle fibres. Passive tension arises from the stretching of the connective tissue beyond its resting length.

Joints
"Joint play" refers to the accessory motion within a joint. The knee (a hinge joint) flexes and extends, but is also capable of a small degree of rotation. A combination of accessory movements, such as rolling and sliding, occurs for it to move.

Convex end

Concave end

Movement occurs with accessory motions

MEASURING MUSCLE STIFFNESS AND FLEXIBLITY

Muscle stiffness is a biomechanical property of muscle tissue that can affect its flexibility and thus how much range of motion you can achieve at a joint. Methods for measuring this have advanced over the years.

The goal of a stretch programme, regardless of the type of stretching used, is typically to improve the range of motion at a particular joint or region of the body. People often seek this out to help prepare for a given activity or sport, such as running, tennis, or strength straining; as part of a physical activity routine; or simply to improve flexibility and reduce muscle stiffness. Measuring the joint range of motion is the most common way of tracking progress.

STIFFNESS VS PERCEIVED TIGHTNESS

Muscle stiffness manifests as a muscle's resistance to stretch, or loss of flexibility. It is influenced by factors such as muscle fibre composition, muscle temperature, and the viscosity, or thickness, of the surrounding tissues. Historically, it has been challenging to measure muscle stiffness due to lack of quality measurement methods. Traditional methods, such as manual palpation – pressing the surface of the body to detect abnormalities – were subjective and relied on the skill level of the examiner. Ultrasound shear wave elastography, which displays tissue stiffness, is a promising new method that can quantify stiffness of a certain soft tissue area.

Perceived muscle tightness refers to the sensation of discomfort or resistance to movement someone feels in a muscle. It is a subjective experience influenced by factors such as muscle fatigue, soreness, and psychological or emotional stress. Perceived muscle tightness may or may not be related to muscle stiffness and it may accompany other connective tissue disorders. Subjective data can be gathered to measure the change in a person's report using questionnaires or visual analogue scales to rate their symptoms. However, because subjective measures of muscle tightness may be influenced by a variety of factors, they should be assessed in conjunction with objective measures to form a comprehensive assessment of muscle function.

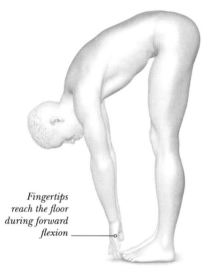

Fingertips reach the floor during forward flexion

BEFORE

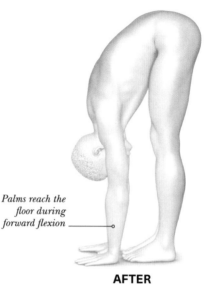

Palms reach the floor during forward flexion

AFTER

SIMPLE ASSESSMENTS
Simple range of motion assessments, like touching your toes, can track changes in flexibility after consistent efforts. Several structures undergo mechanical stress for this motion to occur, including the hamstring muscles, sciatic nerves, and hip joints.

AGE, SEX, AND GENETICS

These three factors can all affect muscle flexibility in different ways. Aging is associated with decreased flexibility, while hormones, joint structure, and genetic composition of muscles, tendons, and connective tissue can also play a role.

Flexibility typically decreases across the lifespan, starting in early adulthood and continuing into old age. This is due to several factors including structural and connective tissue changes, and changes in physical activity. Resistance training can improve function and aerobic exercise benefits cardiovascular health, but basic mobility for daily tasks is still necessary. While not all changes can be improved with flexibility exercises such as joint structure, some can. In particular, flexibility exercises that target the hip flexors and lower limbs have been found to improve gait and balance, and reduce lower back pain in older people. Joint structure can differ between sexes. Females tend to have wider hips and greater flexibility in the lower extremities. However, individual differences in flexibility can also be influenced by factors such as training and lifestyle. Certain genetic differences may lead to differences in joint structure and collagen, which can affect the available range of motion and muscle and tendon properties.

HYPERMOBILITY

Generalized joint hypermobility (GJH) is a hereditary condition that causes an excessive range of motion in the joints. Sometimes this is associated with issues like fibromyalgia (all-over body pain), anxiety, and musculoskeletal injury.

Joint hypermobility is considered a spectrum that ranges from asymptomatic generalized hypermobility to hypermobile Ehlers-Danlos syndromes (EDS), a group of rare, inherited conditions. Research continues to make strides in understanding these conditions, but they are still underappreciated. Symptoms commonly include diffuse pain in load-bearing joints, like the knees, muscle pain, nerve pain, or centrally sensitized pain. Diagnosis and classification are typically made through a series of tests. There is a higher prevalence of hypermobility within some activities, such as ballet dancing, gymnastics, and swimming. With EDS, people may experience joint pain or instability, skin that bruises easily, or symptoms in other body systems such as the digestive, urinary, or cardiovascular systems.

Spectrum of Hypermobility Symptoms

Hypermobility is a spectrum and symptoms are multifactorial per person. The degree of hypermobility does not always correspond to the severity of symptoms.

Peripheral joint hypermobility	Localized joint hypermobility	Generalized joint hypermobility	Symptomatic joint hypermobility
• Hands and feet affected	• One or a few joints affected	• Five or more joints affected	• Hypermobility spectrum disorder and EDS
• Asymptomatic	• Asymptomatic	• Asymptomatic	• Genetic
		• No co-morbidities (other conditions that exist in tandem)	• Musculoskeletal involvement
			• Pain and co-morbidities common

TYPES OF STRETCHING

For the sake of simplicity, stretching options in this book includes static and dynamic stretches, as well as proprioceptive neuromuscular facilitation (PNF) stretches. The choice of stretch used will depend on individual goals and abilities.

DYNAMIC STRETCHING

This type of stretching involves moving a joint through a given range of motion in a controlled manner, and repeating it several times. The two main types of dynamic stretches include active and ballistic stretches.

In dynamic active stretching, you move a joint, or several joints, through their full range of motion to the end ranges, and repeat several times. It is commonly used in a warmup prior to sport or activity, and can be tailored towards activity-specific movements and improving short-term range of motion in preparation for the activity. Dynamic stretching is associated with building strength or performance and has been found to improve running or jumping performance.

Dynamic ballistic stretching (p.42) involves rapid, alternating movements or the momentum of a swinging body segment, like a leg, to lengthen the muscle. Ballistic stretching encourages the stretch reflex, causing the muscles to contract early. Although it may improve performance when done in a warmup, ballistic stretching is not recommended as a standalone treatment for flexibility, because the momentous movement involved increases the risk of injury.

ACTIVE MOVEMENT
Unlike static stretching, which involves holding a stretch in one position, dynamic stretching uses active movements to increase the range of motion of the target. In this Thread the Needle stretch (p.94), the arm repeatedly moves through its full range of motion.

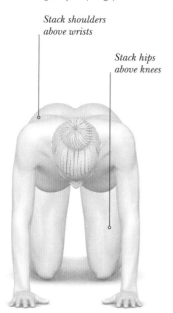

Stack shoulders above wrists

Stack hips above knees

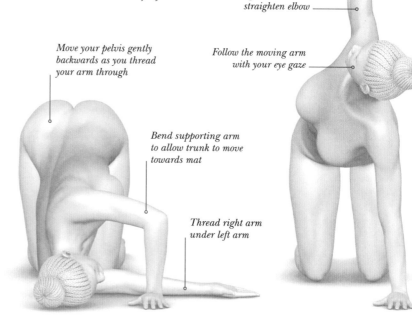

Move your pelvis gently backwards as you thread your arm through

Bend supporting arm to allow trunk to move towards mat

Thread right arm under left arm

Lengthen arm and straighten elbow

Follow the moving arm with your eye gaze

STATIC STRETCHING

This involves holding a position with the muscle on tension to the point of a stretch sensation in order to improve the range of motion. Static stretches can be done with an object, like a wall, or individually.

Static stretching involves holding a stretch for a prolonged period of time, typically from 15 to 30 seconds, and up to 2 minutes. It may be better suited for novices or those who cannot perform more complex dynamic stretches.

Duration spent holding the stretch may vary based on goals. For example, for flexibility gains in larger range of motion positions like the splits, one may need to hold the stretch for longer. The intensity of the stretch may also affect the results of static stretching. Studies have found resistance training can be as effective at increasing joint range of motion as gentle stretching. If static stretching is not working, try strength training, gradually increasing your range of motion.

TIMING
Static stretching, such as this Bent-Knee Calf Stretch (p.168), is typically done when the body is at rest, such as before or after a workout or at the beginning or end of a yoga class.

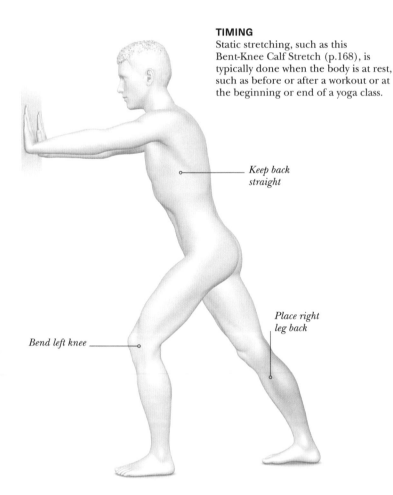

Keep back straight

Place right leg back

Bend left knee

66 99

Static stretching within a warmup that is followed by dynamic activity can improve range of motion without negative effects on subsequent athletic performance.

PROPRIOCEPTIVE NEUROMUSCULAR FACILITATION (PNF)

PNF stretching involves contracting and relaxing stretched muscles to increase range of motion. It may be among the more effective techniques for immediate gains.

PNF stretching was first introduced in the 1940s by Dr Herman Kabat and physical therapists Dorothy Voss and Maggie Knott. It was used as a hands-on treatment approach that enabled clinicians to analyze and assess a patient's movement while facilitating more efficient strategies of functional movement. PNF stretching is used in a variety of settings for different individuals and can yield improvements in flexibility, strength, and power.

Studies have found that PNF stretching can enhance muscular performance when executed in relation to exercise. It can improve muscular performance when performed after or without exercise, but if done beforehand, it may detract from performance.

CONTRACT-RELAX METHOD

The contract-relax (CR) method of PNF stretching involves the target muscle being lengthened and held in a position. Then, the participant contracts the target muscle isometrically (see p.20) to their maximal ability for 3 to 10 seconds. Next, the target muscle is relaxed and passively stretched further. The sequence is repeated 2 to 4 times.

Studies using the CR method have shown improvements in flexibility and range of motion in various muscle groups, including the hamstrings, calves, shoulders, and hip flexors. One study found that the CR method was more effective than static stretching for increasing hamstring flexibility, while another showed that it was more effective than no stretching for improving shoulder range of motion. Of course, long-term carryover of range of motion gains occurs over several weeks of a consistent programme.

Another theory to explain how CR works is autogenic inhibition, a reflex relaxation of a muscle that occurs when it is contracted with a high level of force, to achieve range.

Ballistic stretches

Leg swings that use momentum are an example of ballistic stretching, which involves repetitive motions near the end range of motion. These are typically done with the goal of increasing range of motion and flexibility. Ballistic stretching is generally not recommended for most people but may be used by experienced athletes or qualified professionals.

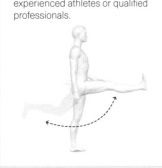

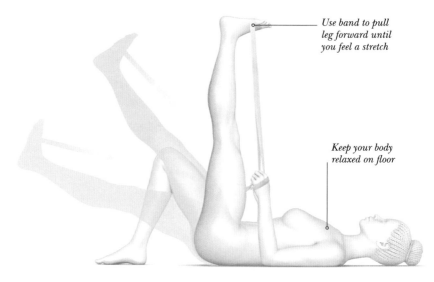

Use band to pull leg forward until you feel a stretch

Keep your body relaxed on floor

CONTRACT-RELAX STRETCH
The contract-relax method can be done with a band or with the help of a partner. Pull the limb into a light to moderate stretch before moving into a contraction.

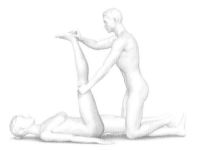

PASSIVE STRETCH: 10 SECS

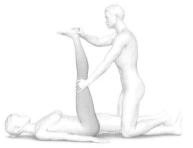

ISOMETRIC HOLD: 6 SECS

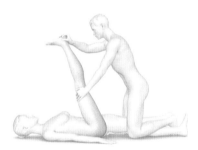

PASSIVE STRETCH: 30 SECS

HOLD-RELAX (HR) METHOD
This is the most common type of PNF stretching. The participant contracts muscles against resistance – in this case a partner – isometrically. Here the quads and hip flexors are passively pushed into a further range of motion for a greater stretch. Both the CR and CRAC methods utilize a passive stretch followed by active tension.

This reflex is activated by golgi tendon organs. The activation of autogenic inhibition helps to enhance muscle relaxation, promoting more flexibility and range of motion.

CR-AGONIST-CONTRACT

With the contract-relax-agonist-contract (CRAC) methods, the same protocol is followed as the CR method. However, another component is added. Instead of passively stretching the target muscle, the participant actively contracts the antagonist muscle to the target muscle, isometrically against resistance, for another given amount of time.

By utilizing the contraction of opposing muscle groups, the CRAC method provides a more comprehensive stretch that targets both agonist and antagonist muscles. This method is also thought to work via autogenic inhibition. By altering the response to the stretch, the participant can move the joint into a greater range of motion. Studies have shown that the CRAC method is effective in improving flexibility in various muscle groups. Some of the muscle groups that have been studied include the hamstrings, hip flexors, adductors, and quadriceps.

The CRAC method may be particularly useful for those recovering from injury or surgery or anyone looking to improve their flexibility. Overall, the CRAC method is another valuable tool for anyone looking to increase their range of motion and flexibility. It is important to note that the various methods of PNF stretching can be intense and should only be performed under the guidance of a trained professional. Additionally, those with certain medical conditions, such as muscle or joint injuries, may need to avoid this kind of stretching or modify the technique to suit their needs.

Types of stretch pros and cons

STRETCH	PROS	CONS
Static	Good for beginners and older adults; improves range of motion at bigger ranges	Time commitment; may detract from performance
Dynamic	May help performance, and doesn't detract from performance; can be done quickly	May not improve larger ranges of motion; has learning curve; needs strength to complete
PNF	Increases range of motion quickly; can improve performance and neuromuscular control	Can be intense and time-consuming; has learning curve

EFFECTS AND BENEFITS OF STRETCHING

Exercise and physical activity have undeniable positive effects on the brain and body. Stretching can be a means of staying active – a practice that society needs as a whole. But the most notable benefits are stretching's effects on range of motion.

THEORIES OF STRETCH ADAPTATION

Regardless of the type of stretching utilized, there are two main theories by which adaptations to stretching occur. Understanding both sensory and mechanical theories can help with making sense of how the body adapts.

All types of stretching have been found to improve range of motion. Scientists have proposed different mechanisms that suggest what happens after muscles are subjected to stretch and how this affects joint flexibility. Many factors play a role in an individual's response to stretching, including the participant's age, experience, and physical characteristics. Nonetheless, science has attempted to explain these mechanisms on the basis of general human physiology.

SENSORY THEORY
The sensory theory proposes that stretch adaptation is primarily a result of changes in stretch tolerance, which is a result of neural adaptations. This includes how golgi tendon organs and muscle spindles play a role in regulating muscle tension during stretching (p.36). The theory suggests that when a muscle is stretched, it stimulates sensory receptors within the muscle and surrounding connective tissue. In the case of reciprocal and autogenic inhibition, the golgi tendon organ helps regulate muscle tension (p.36).

Reciprocal inhibition involves contracting the antagonist muscle group to inhibit the muscle being stretched, while autogenic inhibition involves contracting the muscle being stretched to stimulate the golgi tendon organ and inhibit further contraction. Sensory receptors signal the central nervous system, which modulates the sensitivity of the receptors. With

Did you know?

IN SOME **STRETCHING PROGRAMMES** THAT SPANNED SEVERAL WEEKS, **A JOINT ANGLE INCREASE** OF **17 DEGREES** WAS OBSERVED IN PARTICIPANTS.

66 99

Future research on stretching may explore the effects of different techniques, durations, and frequencies, as well as the mechanisms underlying adaptation.

repeated static stretching, the muscle spindles can adapt and become less sensitive, allowing the muscle to be stretched further without triggering the stretch reflex. Over time, this modulation of sensory input results in an increase in the perceived range of motion. Studies have shown that the sensory theory is evident in single stretching sessions and 3- to-8-week stretching programmes. In these studies, stretch intensity was not increased over time, and the muscle torque, or force, was held constant. The participants were instructed to move until they felt a comfortable stretch and hold, without any additional guidance. Gains in flexibility were observed with as few as 10- to 90-second intervals. In the studies that spanned several weeks, a joint angle increase of 17 degrees was observed within the individual, while the self-reported stretch intensity remained constant.

MECHANICAL THEORY

Muscle is "viscoelastic". This means that muscle-tendon units exhibit both viscous and elastic properties, which allow them to deform and return to their original shape under an applied force, like stretching. When stretching is applied to muscles and connective tissues, they undergo a process called viscoelastic creep, in which they gradually elongate and adapt to the new length.

Underlying theories to explain stretch adaption at the level of the muscle cell are complex. One mechanism involves structural and contractile proteins. While actin and myosin are contractile proteins that generate force during muscle contraction (p.21), titin is a structural protein that provides elasticity and helps maintain the structural integrity of the muscle cell. As the muscle is stretched, the titin molecules are stretched too. This increase in passive tension is

thought to lengthen the muscle cell and contribute to its mechanical adaptation. Another possibility is that stretching can stimulate the production of new connective tissue, such as collagen, which can increase the elasticity and strength of the muscle.

Over time, these changes lead to increased viscoelasticity of the tissues, allowing them to withstand greater forces and elongate more easily. PNF stretching (p.42) is thought to affect both the sensory and mechanical properties of muscle, including the receptors, as well as changes in the viscoelastic properties of muscle tissue.

Overall, the mechanical theory suggests that stretching can lead to physical changes in the muscle tissue, resulting in an increased range of motion and flexibility.

However, there is still debate about the relative importance of the mechanical and sensory theories of stretch adaptation.

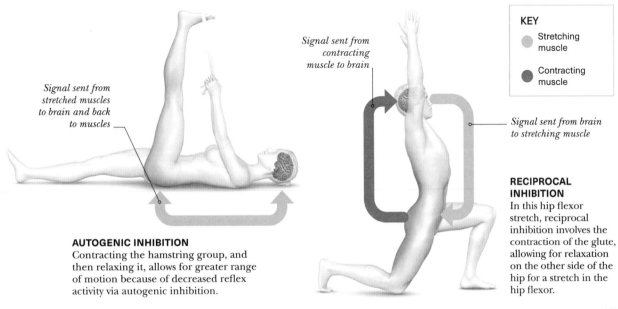

Signal sent from stretched muscles to brain and back to muscles

Signal sent from contracting muscle to brain

KEY
- Stretching muscle
- Contracting muscle

Signal sent from brain to stretching muscle

RECIPROCAL INHIBITION
In this hip flexor stretch, reciprocal inhibition involves the contraction of the glute, allowing for relaxation on the other side of the hip for a stretch in the hip flexor.

AUTOGENIC INHIBITION
Contracting the hamstring group, and then relaxing it, allows for greater range of motion because of decreased reflex activity via autogenic inhibition.

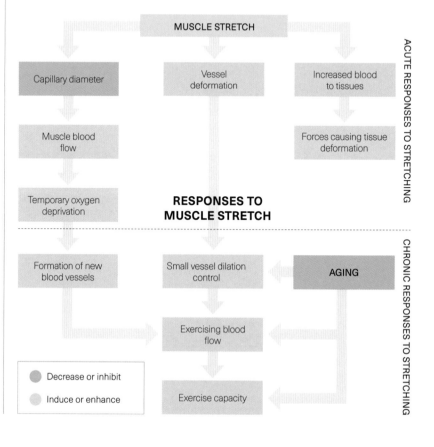

MICROVASCULAR STRUCTURAL BENEFITS

Stretching has been found to improve the structure and function of our smaller blood vessels (microvasculature). It is not yet clear how this varies per individual, or what types of stretching are superior for these effects, but it does pose interesting possibilities about vascular health.

Regular stretching increases the number and density of capillaries in the muscles, leading to improved blood flow and oxygen delivery. This increased blood flow can also help to remove waste products from the muscles more efficiently, improving overall muscle health. Additionally, stretching has been shown to improve the health and function of the endothelium, which is the inner lining of blood vessels. This can improve vascular health, reducing the risk of cardiovascular disease, including high blood pressure.

One study found that stretching may improve microvascular density in older adults, potentially improving blood flow and nutrient delivery to the muscles. Further research is needed to fully understand the mechanisms underlying these microvascular adaptations and their implications.

> **Regular physical activity that includes simple stretching or low-intensity exercise can help aging adults maintain their physical independence.**

Healthy aging

The microvascular adaptations observed in the aging adult population after regular stretching exercises may have significant implications for their overall health and quality of life. By improving blood flow and nutrient delivery to the muscles, stretching may promote muscle regeneration and repair, leading to increased muscle strength and function. Additionally, improved microvascular function may help prevent or mitigate age-related conditions such as cardiovascular disease, cognitive decline, and loss of mobility. These potential benefits suggest that regular stretching can be a simple and effective way for aging adults to maintain their physical health and independence.

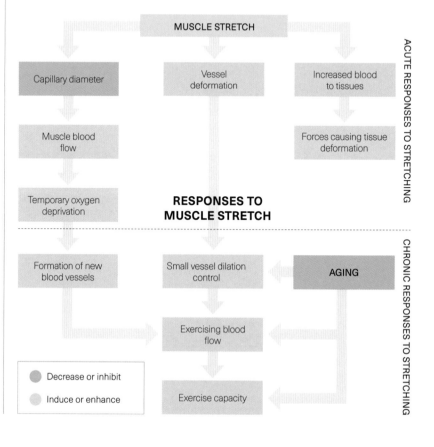

MUSCLE STRETCH

ACUTE RESPONSES TO STRETCHING

Capillary diameter

Vessel deformation

Increased blood to tissues

Muscle blood flow

Forces causing tissue deformation

Temporary oxygen deprivation

RESPONSES TO MUSCLE STRETCH

CHRONIC RESPONSES TO STRETCHING

Formation of new blood vessels

Small vessel dilation control

AGING

Exercising blood flow

Exercise capacity

● Decrease or inhibit

● Induce or enhance

SYSTEM-WIDE BENEFITS

Physical activity, including stretching, benefits the body in a host of ways. The low-intensity nature of stretching, typically aimed at improving joint flexibility, has been shown to positively affect other areas too, including the brain and mental health.

IMPROVES BLOOD PRESSURE

Regular stretching can decrease blood pressure in adults with hypertension. When muscles stretch, blood vessels also stretch and possible changes in microvasculature can affect blood flow.

PROMOTES NEUROPLASTICITY

Stretching and low-intensity exercise increase blood flow and oxygen to the brain, promoting neuroplasticity and cognitive function by enhancing brain-derived neurotrophic factor and other growth factors.

MANAGES WORK-RELATED PAIN

Regular stretch breaks for office workers has been shown to decrease complaints of neck, shoulder, and back pain compared to ergonomic setup alone.

PRESERVES COGNITIVE FUNCTION

Adults over 65 years who participate in regular exercise, including stretching, are more likely to score higher on memory tests and be at a reduced risk for dementia.

IMPROVES MOBILITY

Stretching can help retain and improve flexibility, which can have a positive effect on function throughout the lifespan, particularly in older adults.

IMPROVES NEUROMUSCULAR CONTROL AND FUNCTION

Using the muscles regularly in dynamic stretches, including PNF techniques, can improve how they function and control movement.

IMPROVES MENTAL HEALTH

Studies have found positive effects on mood, depression, and anxiety levels after engaging in stretching and low-intensity exercise, as well as improved serotonin uptake in the brain.

ENCOURAGES SLEEP QUALITY

Regular stretching can improve sleep quality, particularly in older adults with cognitive and sleep disturbances.

IMPROVES MOOD AND COGNITION

Acute stretching improve mood states, which may contribute to a positive effect on cognitive performance in physically inactive people.

REDUCES SEDENTARY BEHAVIOUR

Participating in a regular stretching programme allows a means for low-intensity exercise, thus reducing sedentary behaviour and the negative effects that accompany it.

STRETCHING AND MAINTAINING FITNESS

Physical activity is a key component of a healthy lifestyle, and removing barriers to exercise to increase participation is at the forefront of global health initiatives. Evidence to support how stretching plays a role in physical fitness has evolved over the years.

THE IMPORTANCE OF FITNESS

Strong evidence supports the idea that regular physical activity and exercise are essential for maintaining and improving physical fitness. Physical components gained, like strength and endurance, can maximize health and wellbeing.

Physical fitness is a state of wellbeing that encompasses both physical and mental health. It is the ability to perform daily activities with ease, without undue fatigue, and with enough energy to engage in leisure activities.

It includes several attributes, such as cardiorespiratory endurance, muscular strength and endurance, flexibility, body composition, and other skills and aptitudes such as agility, balance, coordination, power, reaction time, and speed. Physical fitness can be achieved through regular physical activity that is tailored to individual goals and needs. Flexibility training, through stretching, takes commitment and time because the body takes time to adapt. Range of motion is one way to measure flexibility; it can also be measured by how you tolerate ranges of motion, the quality of your movement, and personal experience in achieving them.

With this in mind, you can be empowered to supplement your physical activity routine with stretching and mobility exercises that are relevant to your goals, and positively contribute to your movement and fitness journey over your lifespan.

GOALS AND ROUTINES

Setting goals when embarking on a programme can improve physical fitness, and implementing stretching within training programmes for specific goals can help maximize outcomes. However, adherence is key for any physical change. When setting goals, consider factors like current abilities, time or environmental constraints, and training intent, for example, sports or general function.

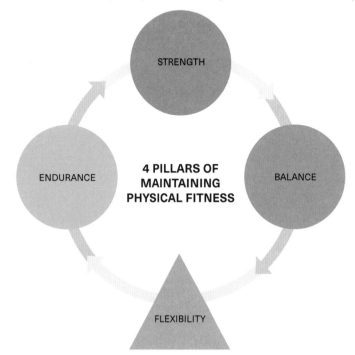

STRENGTH

ENDURANCE

4 PILLARS OF MAINTAINING PHYSICAL FITNESS

BALANCE

FLEXIBILITY

Strength

Muscular strength is the ability of a muscle or muscle group to generate maximal force against a resistance through a full range of motion. Strength can improve bone density, blood sugar regulation, blood pressure, and cardiovascular health. Basic exercises typically involve multi-joint movements targeting major muscle groups. A qualified personal trainer or exercise specialist can assist with this.

Programming Tips

Target all major muscle groups at least twice per week.

Do 1 to 3 sets of 8 to 12 repetitions at a weight that is 60-80 per cent of your 1-rep maximum.

- **Lower body exercise ideas:** squats, lunges, deadlifts.
- **Upper body exercise ideas:** bench press, overhead press, bicep curls, tricep extensions, front raises.
- **Core exercise ideas:** planks, sit ups.

Balance

Balance is the ability to maintain or return the body's centre of mass within the base of support in any given sensory environment. Balance exercises can help improve proprioception and neuromuscular control, reducing the risk of falls and improving functional ability. Incorporating balance training in a well-rounded fitness programme may include the use of different surfaces or unilateral exercises.

Programming Tips

Incorporate a variety of exercises to challenge different sensory and motor systems. Perform in a safe environment with proper supervision.

Exercise ideas: stand on one leg, single-leg squats, stand on an unstable surface like foam pad. Challenge the sensory system by opening or closing the eyes, or performing head turns on one leg.

Flexibility

Flexibility is the ability of a joint or series of joints to move through a full, non-restricted range of motion (ROM). Flexibility can be improved through regular stretching exercises that target the major muscle groups. Stretching can be done for general fitness, before exercise, or as part of sports training.

Programming Tips

General fitness: Do 2–3 sets of 15–30 seconds of static stretching, 2–3 days per week

Before exercise: Do 2–4 sets of 10–15 dynamic repetitions. If opting for static stretches, follow up with dynamic activity.

Sports: These flexibility programmes may be done for longer durations and at higher intensities. Do 10–15 minute programmes, 3–4 days per week.

Endurance

Endurance is the ability to sustain physical activity or exercise for prolonged periods of time. Endurance is an important component of physical fitness and is commonly assessed through measures such as maximal oxygen uptake (VO2 max) or the ability to maintain a given pace or power output over a specified duration. This may include aerobic, anaerobic, or muscular endurance.

Programming Tips

- Include regular, progressive training.
- Gradually increase the duration, intensity, or volume of exercise over time.
- Allow adequate rest and recovery between sessions.
- Utilize interval training.

Aerobic training ideas: running, cycling, swimming.
Anaerobic training ideas: sprinting, weightlifting.
Muscular training ideas: bodyweight exercises, plyometric training, isometric exercises, high-repetition weight training, circuit training.

STRETCHING FOR INJURY RECOVERY AND PAIN RELIEF

Pain is complex and injuries are multifactorial, and the role of stretching to address each depends on many things. As stretching has historically been sought out as a treatment for athletic preparation and pain relief, it's worth reviewing the basics here.

GENERAL INJURY REDUCTION

Injuries occur for many reasons and while we can't prevent every injury, we can aim to reduce the risks. Injuries can result from a variety of factors, such as overuse, so injury prevention and rehabilitation strategies should be tailored to the individual and the sport, activity, or injury.

Different types of stretching are preferred for different activities and while stretching is commonly done before exercise and can increase flexibility, its relevance to preventing musculoskeletal injury is currently not well understood.

Evidence continues to encourage a multi-modal approach to reducing injury risk – stretching alone is not sufficient to prevent all kinds of injuries. Instead, aspects like load management, proper sleep, recovery, nutrition, strength training, and activity preparation should be prioritized. Stretching can be used as an adjunct to a complete, individualized training programme tailored to a specific activity in order for injury reduction efforts to be most successful.

Stretching can be beneficial for reducing certain types of pain, such as chronic lower back pain. However, any stretching to address injury or pain should be performed in a safe and controlled manner, and caution should be taken to avoid overstretching or causing further injury.

Injury risk profile

Why do injuries occur? A complex combination of factors contributes to each person's personal injury risk profile. Injury risk increases or decreases depending on the interaction between internal and external factors.

INTERNAL/PERSONAL	EXTERNAL/ENVIROMENTAL
Biological These internal risk factors represent the physical and physiological characteristics of a person. They include elements like age, size, fatigue levels, prior injury, fitness levels, training programme, and biomechanical factors.	**Physical** These refer to the physical environment surrounding the participation of the individual in exercise: elements such as weather, facilities available, terrain, and equipment. These characteristics are independent of the person.
Psychological These internal risk factors represent all the different mental characteristics at play in a person. They include elements such as life and life event stressors, type of mood, coping skills, beliefs, and attitudes. Together, all these factors combine to affect mental wellbeing.	**Sociocultural** These risk factors refer to external influences such as the quality of officiating in a given sport, coaching, and social pressures to exercise or perform. These are characteristics that embody the sociocultural environment in which the person is situated.

66 99

Injury risk changes based on the interaction of internal and external factors affecting an individual.

MUSCULOSKELETAL INJURIES

This segment will explain the differences between common injury types. Injuries can be daunting, but learning the physiology of the body's structures can help in honouring the body's needs to adapt and heal.

Musculoskeletal injuries are a common type of injury that can affect the body's bones, tendons, ligaments, muscles, and other soft tissues. Recovery times depend on factors like the severity of the injury, the tissues involved, and the individual.

Injury rehabilitation requires an individualized plan designed by a qualified professional to support tissue recovery to regain function, like returning to running or being able to walk again after a broken ankle. It is common for tissues to lose flexibility after periods of immobilization. When certain options for exercise or resistance training are not yet attainable, guided stretching exercises or other low-intensity movements can help to restore joint range of motion. Regardless of injury type, common goals of injury rehabilitation include managing pain and swelling, restoring joint range of motion, proprioception training, strengthening and neuromuscular control, and a plan to get back to normal activities. While stretching may be included in a rehabilitation programme, it should always be in addition to a more complete plan.

Strain vs sprain

These terms refer to injuries, but in different structures. A strain is an excessive stretch or tear in the muscle belly or tendon, while sprains occur in ligaments or joint capsules.

- **Strains:** Excessive force or tension in the muscle beyond its tolerance. **Examples:** quadriceps strain, hamstring strain, biceps strain

- **Sprains:** Joint is forced past its normal anatomical limits, resulting in injury to the ligaments. **Examples:** ACL, MCL, LCL sprains, ankle sprain

- **Grading:** On a scale from I to III.

TYPES OF INJURIES

Acute, chronic, and overuse injuries are different ways to describe musculoskeletal injury patterns. Acute injuries result from sudden and forceful impact or trauma. These injuries often cause immediate symptoms and may require immediate medical attention. Examples of acute injuries include fractures, sprains, and strains. Chronic injuries persist for a long time or recur frequently, like lower back pain. Overuse injuries result from repetitive stress or strain on a specific part of the body over a period of time. Examples of overuse injuries include tendinopathy and stress fractures.

The management and treatment of these different types of injuries may vary, but teatment generally involves controlling pain and inflammation, physical therapy, surgery, or another plan of care. For chronic and overuse injuries, treatment may involve modifications to activity or lifestyle, as well as rehabilitation and management of underlying conditions.

Ligament sprain
Graded from I-III; possible immobilization, gradual return to activities.

Ligament tear
Can be partial or complete; may require surgical repair.

Tendon injury
Overuse or acute; requires rehabilitation or surgical intervention.

Fracture
Break in the bone; likely immobilization, possible surgical repair.

Muscle

Ligament

Tendon

COMMON MUSCULOSKELETAL INJURIES

Muscle strain
Graded from I-III; compression, elevation, rehabilitation.

Dislocation
Bone forced out of place; requires prompt medical attention.

OPTIONS FOR PAIN MANAGEMENT

Physical activity can be an effective form of pain management, as can stretching – especially in the context of musculoskeletal pain. Regular exercise may even reduce the need for pain medication. Since pain is complex, there are many options to help treat it.

Studies have shown that regular physical activity can significantly reduce pain and improve function in individuals with chronic pain, as well as lowering healthcare costs and reducing the need for pain medications. Stretching, in particular, has been shown to reduce pain and improve mobility in those with all kinds of lower back pain, knee osteoarthritis, and chronic neck pain. Stretching can help improve flexibility, reduce stiffness, and alleviate pain in individuals with various musculoskeletal conditions. However, it's important to work with a healthcare provider to develop an individualized pain management plan that takes into account the specific type and severity of the pain, as well as individual health and lifestyle factors.

A SIGNAL FROM THE BODY

Pain is a signal from the body that may or may not always indicate tissue damage. Some other successful pain relief approaches include mindfulness therapy, breathwork, and cognitive behavioural therapy (CBT). Mindfulness refers to being present with an open and non-judgmental attitude. Breathwork involves using breathing techniques to promote relaxation and reduce stress. It can help decrease pain by reducing stress and tension. CBT can help change the way individuals think and respond to pain. These approaches may be used alone or in combination with other pain management strategies, such as medication or physical therapy.

MOVEMENT AND PAIN RELIEF
Pain is a personal experience influenced by many variables. There are several non-pharmacological ways to approach pain relief, including regular low-intensity exercise.

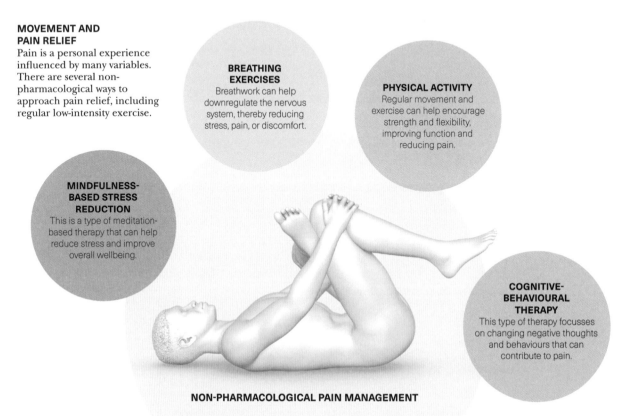

BREATHING EXERCISES
Breathwork can help downregulate the nervous system, thereby reducing stress, pain, or discomfort.

PHYSICAL ACTIVITY
Regular movement and exercise can help encourage strength and flexibility, improving function and reducing pain.

MINDFULNESS-BASED STRESS REDUCTION
This is a type of meditation-based therapy that can help reduce stress and improve overall wellbeing.

COGNITIVE-BEHAVIOURAL THERAPY
This type of therapy focusses on changing negative thoughts and behaviours that can contribute to pain.

NON-PHARMACOLOGICAL PAIN MANAGEMENT

IMPORTANCE OF BREATHING

Breathing not only plays a role in stress reduction and vital signs, but the muscles which are used to breathe can contribute to how we move, and to pressure management within the abdominal cavity.

The primary breathing muscles are in the diaphragm and the intercostals. The diaphragm is key, as it contracts and flattens to pull air into the lungs. The intercostal muscles help to expand the chest and increase lung capacity during inhalation.

The accessory breathing muscles can assist with breathing when the primary muscles are strained, such as during situations like exercise or if the primary muscles are weak due to illness or injury. These muscles include the abdominal muscles, and the sternocleidomastoid, scalenes, and trapezius muscles in the neck and shoulders. These muscles can be helpful, but relying on them excessively for breathing can lead to strain and fatigue.

BREATHING MECHANICS

Quiet breathing refers to the normal, automatic breathing that occurs when the body is at rest. The diaphragm and intercostal muscles work together to expand the chest and pull air into the lungs, without the need for conscious effort or control. Active breathing, on the other hand, involves more conscious control of the breathing process. This may include techniques such as deep breathing or belly breathing.

> " "
>
> *Breathing exercises that are geared towards relaxation can be a useful tool for improving mobility and reducing pain in the neck, chest, and shoulders.*

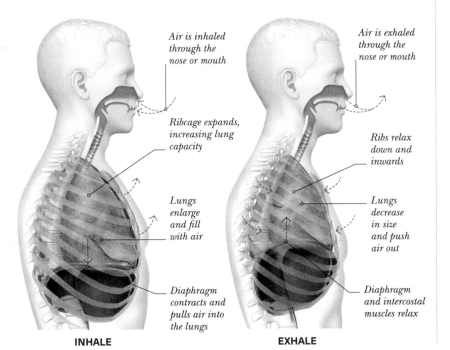

Air is inhaled through the nose or mouth

Ribcage expands, increasing lung capacity

Lungs enlarge and fill with air

Diaphragm contracts and pulls air into the lungs

INHALE

Air is exhaled through the nose or mouth

Ribs relax down and inwards

Lungs decrease in size and push air out

Diaphragm and intercostal muscles relax

EXHALE

CONSCIOUS CONTROL

Conscious control of the breath during activities can reduce muscle tension and anxiety, making it a useful tool in pain management. In diaphragmatic breathing, we use the dome-shaped diaphragm muscle under the lungs to get more air into our lungs, and more oxygen to the brain. This slows the heartbeat and lowers blood pressure.

STRETCHING AND HEALTHY AGING

Skeletal muscle mass and strength naturally decline with age, in a process called sarcopenia. This decrease in muscle mass and strength can lead to reduced mobility. Staying physically active can help maintain full function and independence.

MUSCLE PROPERTIES THROUGH THE LIFESPAN

Aging skeletal muscle undergoes several changes, including a decrease in the size and number of muscle fibres, the ability to generate force quickly, and a decrease in joint flexibility. All of these aspects have the potential to affect normal daily function.

Several changes occur within skeletal muscle that contribute to the age-related decline in muscle mass and strength. First, there is a progressive loss of muscle fibres, and a loss in overall muscle strength. There is also a decline in the number and function of motor neurons that control muscle contraction. A decrease in the rate of muscle protein synthesis and an increase in breakdown can contribute to a loss of muscle mass over time. Metabolic properties, such as a decrease in energy metabolism, can also negatively affect muscle function.

Tendon properties also change with age. They become stiffer and less compliant, which can negatively affect joint mobility. This is because tendons are responsible for transmitting forces from the muscle to the bone and the increased stiffness can interfere with this process.

The combination of changes in muscle and tendon properties with age can negatively impact physical function and mobility, and resulting falls can have a significant impact on an older person's quality of life.

Sarcopenia is a progressive, age-related syndrome causing the

Sarcopenia

This term describes the loss of muscle mass, strength, and function in aging skeletal muscle. Mitochondria within the muscle also degenerate with age and inactivity. To prevent and manage sarcopenia, it's important to stay active, eat well, and practise resistance training.

YOUNG AGE/PHYSICALLY ACTIVE	OLD AGE/PHYSICALLY ACTIVE	OLD AGE/SEDENTARY

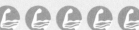

Muscle
Skeletal muscle has normal mass, strength, and function. It easily builds in response to an appropriate stimulus.

Muscle
With adequate activity, skeletal muscles can still maintain a certain level of strength and mass which encourages function.

Muscle
Skeletal muscle has decreased mass and strength, which negatively impacts function.

Mitochondria
Young, active muscle has higher numbers of mitochondria, responsible for energy production and adequate skeletal function.

Mitochondria
Mitochondrial health and function are maintained with exercise, allowing for continued energy production.

Mitochondria
Aging, sedentary skeletal muscle has decreased mitochondrial content and function, with more decline than production.

loss of skeletal strength, often occurring before loss of muscle mass and function.

However, it can be prevented, treated, and managed, depending on its cause and duration.

Despite all these changes, regular exercise can help slow down the age-related decline in muscle and tendon properties. Resistance training and other weightbearing exercises can help maintain and improve muscle mass and strength, while stimulating tendon growth. With training, and practice, older adults can still participate in all kinds of exercise safely.

MUSCLE ADAPTS

Although aging leads to a decline in muscle mass and strength, skeletal muscle still retains the ability to adapt with age, provided it is exposed to the appropriate training stimulus.

Research suggests that older muscles are just as responsive to exercise as younger muscles, although the rate and magnitude of the response may be reduced.

Static and dynamic stretching, as shown in this book, have been found to improve muscle flexibility and joint range of motion in older adults. Adequate protein intake is also essential for promoting muscle protein synthesis and hypertrophy (muscle gain) in response to a regular exercise programme.

In short, while stretching can have benefits for maintaining flexibility and joint range of motion in aging skeletal muscle, it should be combined with other types of exercise, such as resistance training, and with consideration for adequate nutrition, for optimal muscle health and function.

PHYSICAL ACTIVITY REQUIREMENTS

Physical inactivity is a major risk factor for many chronic diseases and deaths worldwide. To try to rectify this, the World Health Organization (WHO) has created exercise guidelines.

It is recommended that adults aged 18 to 64 years should engage in at least 150 minutes of moderate-intensity aerobic physical activity throughout the week, or at least 75 minutes of vigorous-intensity aerobic physical activity throughout the week, or an equivalent combination of both. Adults should also engage in resistance training to strengthen muscles at least twice per week. These activities should address all major muscle groups, like the hip flexors, knee extensors, and shoulder muscles, and be performed at a moderate to high intensity. Some physical activity is better than none –

individuals should aim to be as physically active as possible within their own abilities and circumstances. Those who are sedentary should gradually increase physical activity levels over time, in consultation with their healthcare provider if needed.

The goal of increasing physical activity is to reduce the burden of chronic diseases, improve mental health and wellbeing, and enhance the overall quality of life globally. The guidelines recognize that physical activity can be brought into everyday life in a variety of ways, and that people can choose activities safe for their level of fitness and ability.

PHYSICAL ACTIVITY GUIDELINES
A bout of moderate or vigorous intensity physical activity, or both, is recommended for older adults throughout the week.

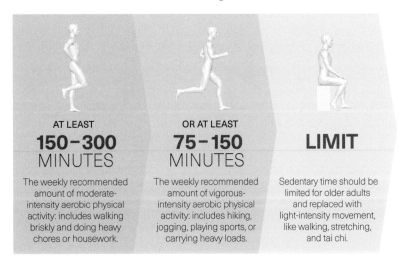

AT LEAST	OR AT LEAST	
150–300 MINUTES	**75–150** MINUTES	**LIMIT**
The weekly recommended amount of moderate-intensity aerobic physical activity: includes walking briskly and doing heavy chores or housework.	The weekly recommended amount of vigorous-intensity aerobic physical activity: includes hiking, jogging, playing sports, or carrying heavy loads.	Sedentary time should be limited for older adults and replaced with light-intensity movement, like walking, stretching, and tai chi.

STRETCHING GUIDELINES FOR OLDER PEOPLE

With age, it becomes more important than ever to stay active. Resistance and aerobic exercises are two modes of physical activity that should be included in an exercise routine to maintain function. Stretching can help to make physical activity more accessible and enjoyable for older adults, which can in turn promote overall health and wellbeing.

When it comes to older adults, maintaining function for daily activities and reducing risk of falls or injuries is a priority. Exercise recommendations include reducing sedentary time and replacing it with low-intensity movement, like stretching or tai chi. Upper body flexibility is important for activities like getting dressed and reaching for objects, while lower body flexibility is important for walking and bending. Stretches targeting joints used in daily life should be included.

Of course, older adults can still and should train for more rigorous movement goals. Movement should be varied and emphasize balance and strength training, preferably at moderate or higher intensities. This is recommended on three or more days per week, in tandem with stretching programmes, to improve functional capacity and reduce the risk of falls.

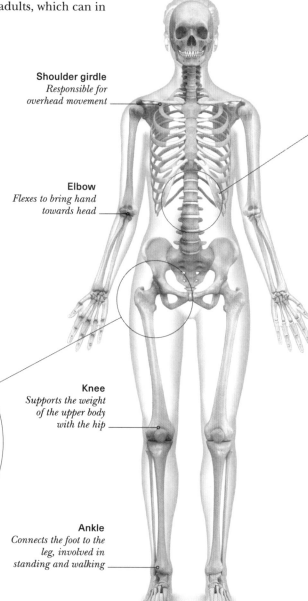

Shoulder girdle
Responsible for overhead movement

Elbow
Flexes to bring hand towards head

Knee
Supports the weight of the upper body with the hip

Ankle
Connects the foot to the leg, involved in standing and walking

ANTERIOR VIEW

Psoas major
Primary hip flexor

Iliacus
Joined with the psoas, adds to hip flexion

adductor longus
Contributes to hip flexion, stabilizes pelvis during movement

Hip flexors

Stretching the hip flexors and extensors has been shown to improve gait in older adults. This is especially important to reduce risk of falls and maintain functional mobility and independence.

Trunk muscles

These contribute to core stability, posture, and balance. Maintaining strength and flexibility here with regular exercise like Pilates and tai chi can support mobility and quality of life.

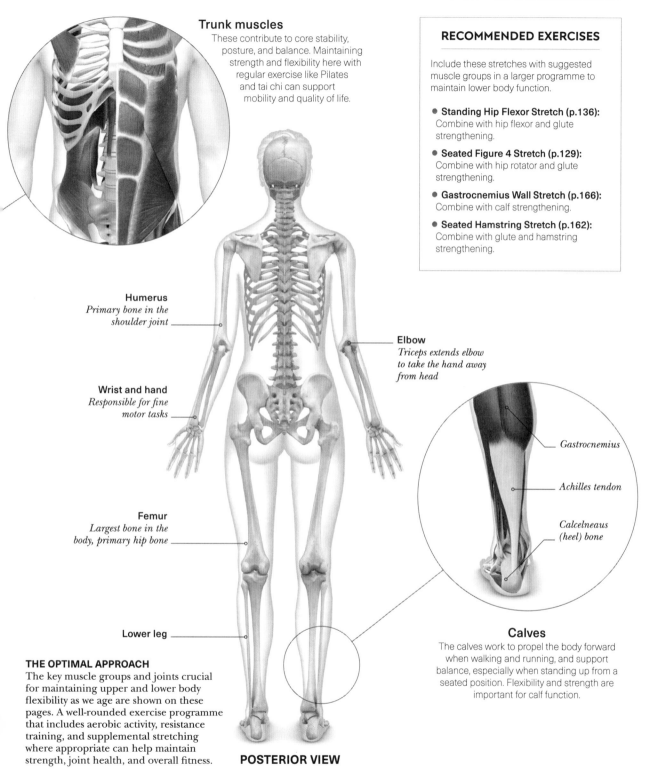

RECOMMENDED EXERCISES

Include these stretches with suggested muscle groups in a larger programme to maintain lower body function.

- **Standing Hip Flexor Stretch (p.136):** Combine with hip flexor and glute strengthening.
- **Seated Figure 4 Stretch (p.129):** Combine with hip rotator and glute strengthening.
- **Gastrocnemius Wall Stretch (p.166):** Combine with calf strengthening.
- **Seated Hamstring Stretch (p.162):** Combine with glute and hamstring strengthening.

Humerus
Primary bone in the shoulder joint

Elbow
Triceps extends elbow to take the hand away from head

Wrist and hand
Responsible for fine motor tasks

Gastrocnemius

Achilles tendon

Calcelneaus (heel) bone

Femur
Largest bone in the body, primary hip bone

Lower leg

THE OPTIMAL APPROACH

The key muscle groups and joints crucial for maintaining upper and lower body flexibility as we age are shown on these pages. A well-rounded exercise programme that includes aerobic activity, resistance training, and supplemental stretching where appropriate can help maintain strength, joint health, and overall fitness.

Calves

The calves work to propel the body forward when walking and running, and support balance, especially when standing up from a seated position. Flexibility and strength are important for calf function.

POSTERIOR VIEW

WHEN NOT TO STRETCH

It is important to be aware of general precautions and contraindications to stretching. However, you should always consult a trained professional for guidance on treatment of specific injuries and medical conditions.

STRETCH PRECAUTIONS

Stretching has been proven to positively affect joint range of motion and flexibility, but emphasizing safe practices is key to minimizing the risk of injury or exacerbating existing health conditions. By following appropriate precautions and seeking professional guidance, individuals can improve their flexibility and function while reducing the risk of injury or harm.

There are situations where not all stretching is appropriate and it should be administered by a trained professional. These include acute injuries, such as a muscle strain or sprain, joint instability, or after a recent joint replacement surgery. Other incidences include an open wound, joint dislocation, or infection. Stretching is not likely to be immediately recommended for these cases as pain management or following other protocols are prioritized.

In some cases, immobilization or other joint precautions are in place to protect the affected area. These precautions may be temporary, but are there to honour tissue healing.

Other situations where caution is warranted are with non-acute conditions or pregnancy. For example, individuals who have chronic pain or conditions such as osteoporosis or rheumatoid arthritis may need to modify or avoid certain stretches to prevent injury or discomfort. Stretching throughout pregnancy may warrant modified positions. A trained healthcare professional or qualified coach should be consulted to ease any health concerns or conditions that may impact your ability to stretch safely or exercise effectively.

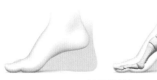

NORMAL

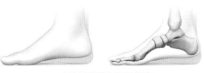

HALLUX LIMITUS

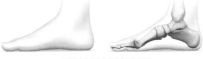

HALLUX RIGIDUS

BIG TOE DISORDERS
With normal big toe range of motion, you can easily flex the joint. With hallux limitus, the toe is stiff but can move slightly; with hallux rigidus, the toe has virtually no movement at all.

JOINT CHANGES
Joint changes can affect range of motion by altering the structure and function of the bones. For example, osteoarthritis can contribute to the loss of cartilage and the development of bone spurs, which can limit the joint's ability to move smoothly and freely. Changes to the joint capsule or surrounding soft tissues can also limit the range of motion. Proprioceptive feedback from the joint may change, leading to decreased sensory input and impaired control of movement. Care should be taken while stretching or attempting to gain motion in the presence of these.

For example, hallux limitus is a condition where there is limited range of motion and stiffness in the big toe joint, often caused by the development of osteoarthritis or other joint surface changes. While there may be some stiffness or discomfort, the toe is still able to move to some degree. Hallux rigidus is a more severe form of hallux limitus, where there is little to no range of motion in the big toe joint, partially due to advanced joint surface changes or bony growths

Hip impingment

Hip joints vary in shape and size. Some variations can lead to femoroacetabular hip impingement (FAI), where the ball pinches against the socket, causing pain, stiffness, and limited range of motion. Rehabilitation aims to improve hip stability, neuromuscular control, strength, range of motion, and movement patterns.

Bones fit perfectly together

NORMAL

Bone overgrowth on femoral head, which is not perfectly round

CAM

Hip socket and femoral head

SUPERIOR VIEW

Bone overcoverage of the rim of the socket

PINCER

Bone overgrowth on both sides of femoral head

MIXED

that limit movement and cause pain and discomfort.

Some signs that may indicate joint-related limitations in range of motion include:

- Sharp, dull, or achy pain, and may be worse with movement.

- May feel tight or difficult to move, worse in the morning or after prolonged periods of inactivity.

- Local pain or inflammation causing pain or stiffness.

- Decreased range of motion – can be mild or severe.

- Pain or catching, with popping or clicking.

STRUCTURAL ANATOMY

Sometimes natural variations in joint structure, called morphologies,

can limit range of motion and contribute to pain or injury if overloaded or stressed. These variations can occur in different regions of the body and can range from relatively common to rare.

In the hip joint, for example, cam and pincer morphologies are two common variations that can affect range of motion, especially flexion and rotation (see above).

Acetabular retroversion occurs when the acetabulum (socket) is pointed towards the back of the pelvis, leading to decreased range of motion between the femur and the acetabulum. Acetabular anteversion occurs when the acetabulum is oriented towards the front of the pelvis. These variations can be present and asymptomatic. If they are causing limitations, seek treatment options like physical therapy from a healthcare provider.

Safety and limits

If joint structure is a limiting factor, flexibility may be limited as a result and gains may be limited. It's important to honour these limitations and recognize when not to push aggressively into range with activity, such as stretching. Consider these exercise tips:

- **Sharp, lingering aches** or pains indicate aggravation.

- **Avoid pushing aggressively** into end-range of motion.

- **Maximize strength** in the available range.

- **Gradually increase** physical activity and exercise intensity.

- **Modify stretch positions** for comfort – many of the stretches featured in this book include variations that modifiy their intensity and provide both seated and standing options.

- **Ask a trained professional** for guidance.

STRETCH
EXERCISES

This section offers a clear, step-by-step guide to set up and execute a carefully chosen set of stretch exercises. They are arranged by body area, so you can be sure all parts – even your wrists – will be stretched. With no need for equipment, stretching is available to everyone, and there are many ways to include stretching in your physical activity routine. Modifications and safety notes throughout allow people of all levels to upgrade their mobility and flexibility training without fear of strain or injury .

INTRODUCTION TO THE EXERCISES

Stretching has evolved hugely over time, in both how it is performed and in our understanding of it. Research continues to study the effects of stretching on the body and how it relates to our functions as humans and the activities we choose to partake in. This is simply an introduction.

Before starting on your stretching journey, it's important to understand a few factors. Once you have mastered the technique for a static stretch, try to hold it for 15 to 30 seconds, and up to a maximum of 60 seconds when you become accustomed to it, to gain the optimal benefit in flexibility. However, for greater ranges of motion and training (such as in gymnastics), increased intensity and duration of stretches may be required.

As well as the stretches in this book, full-range resistance training is also a viable option for improving joint range of motion and plays an important role in tissue tolerance. The best advice is to aim to stay as physically active as you can throughout your lifespan.

INTENTS AND GOALS

The stretches you choose to do will depend on your goals. You have the option to stretch for basic functional mobility or train for flexibility. You can use dynamic stretches to supplement your current preferred activity, be it running or playing soccer. You may choose to include static stretches to increase the flexibility needed for a specific sport, or perhaps you'd just like to explore movement in general. Realize that there may be days when a range of motion feels or seems different from the day before, or days when it seems better. Appreciate the sensations and quality of movement along the way. The body needs time and repeated efforts to adapt. How you choose to use this book is up to you. The purpose is to supply you with the knowledge of what is known today, and remove barriers to exercise and physical activity.

STRETCH BOTH SIDES

Many of the exercises that follow, such as the Standing Half Moon (p.92), explain how to stretch one side of the body (left or right). With each of these, it's important to repeat the same stretch on the other side of the body.

Equipment

Many stretches can be done without the use of equipment. But not only can small equipment help with comfort, it can also help push stretch intensity or contribute to gains with active stretches. Some examples to enhance your workout include resistance bands, yoga blocks, exercise mats, or a bench. Yoga blocks are great for modifying the depth of stretches or reducing the reach necessary. Resistance bands can be added to active movements, such as wall rotations. Some of the exercises featured in this book will involve these.

- **Resistance bands:** These typically come in long loops or single strips. They may be added to various stretches for a strength component.

- **Yoga blocks:** Blocks or bolsters can help modify the range of motion and offer support.

- **Exercise mat:** Mats offer comfort on a hard surface, and come in various thicknesses.

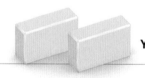

RESISTANCE BAND

YOGA BLOCKS

EXERCISE MAT

DIFFERENT STRETCH DISCIPLINES

Each type of stretch discipline has its own history, principles, focus, and approach. Some of the following stretches reflect these disciplines, but there are also new stretches you may not have come across before.

Some common types of disciplines that involve the use of stretching include yoga, Pilates, or tai chi. There are also other mobility programmes that utilize their own philosophies, guidelines, and intents. Many stretches featured across these disciplines may share names or vary slightly.

For example, Child's Pose (p.78) is practised in yoga and in many other fitness settings. Cat Cow (p.74) is also performed across different disciplines. These may be included in a larger sequence of yoga postures and can be combined with other postures, breathing techniques, and meditation practices.

Overall, the differences between stretching disciplines reflect the diverse range of goals and preferences of individuals who engage in physical activity, as well as the specific needs and requirements of different types of athletes or populations.

CHOOSING THE RIGHT EXERCISE

Choosing the right exercise will depend on factors like goals, physical abilities, and any health conditions or injuries. Guidelines are provided, but normal movement variation exists. You can choose to perform stretches in areas you wish

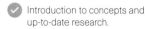

This book is about:
The goal of this book is to help educate about current concepts in stretching, remove barriers to physical activity, and encourage movement exploration.

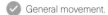

- ✓ Introduction to concepts and up-to-date research.
- ✓ General movement.
- ✓ A resource to appreciate movement and your body's abilities within movement.

This book is not about:
The purpose of this book is not to replace medical advice or be a means of self-treatment. Always ask a professional for individual concerns.

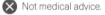

- ✗ Not medical advice.
- ✗ Individual limitations may affect performance of exercises. Pain and injury should always be properly assessed.

to become more flexible, or to support a specific type of physical activity. Many stretches may have a unilateral or asymmetrical position that may be done on both sides.

Remember that when you embark on a stretch programme, including other types of exercise is key for the best outcomes. While some discomfort is normal, it should be temporary. If pain persists or you have specific health concerns, consult a qualified professional, such as a physical therapist or personal trainer.

THE COMMON DENOMINATOR
Stretching can be found in all kinds of activities such as yoga, Pilates, and general fitness training. While their individual intents and philosophies may differ, movement is the common theme, central to all.

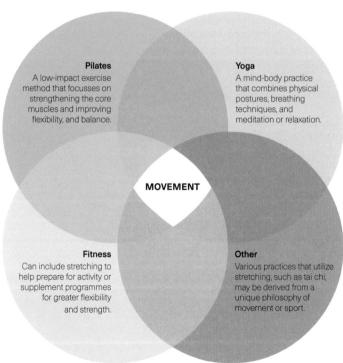

Pilates
A low-impact exercise method that focusses on strengthening the core muscles and improving flexibility, and balance.

Yoga
A mind-body practice that combines physical postures, breathing techniques, and meditation or relaxation.

MOVEMENT

Fitness
Can include stretching to help prepare for activity or supplement programmes for greater flexibility and strength.

Other
Various practices that utilize stretching, such as tai chi, may be derived from a unique philosophy of movement or sport.

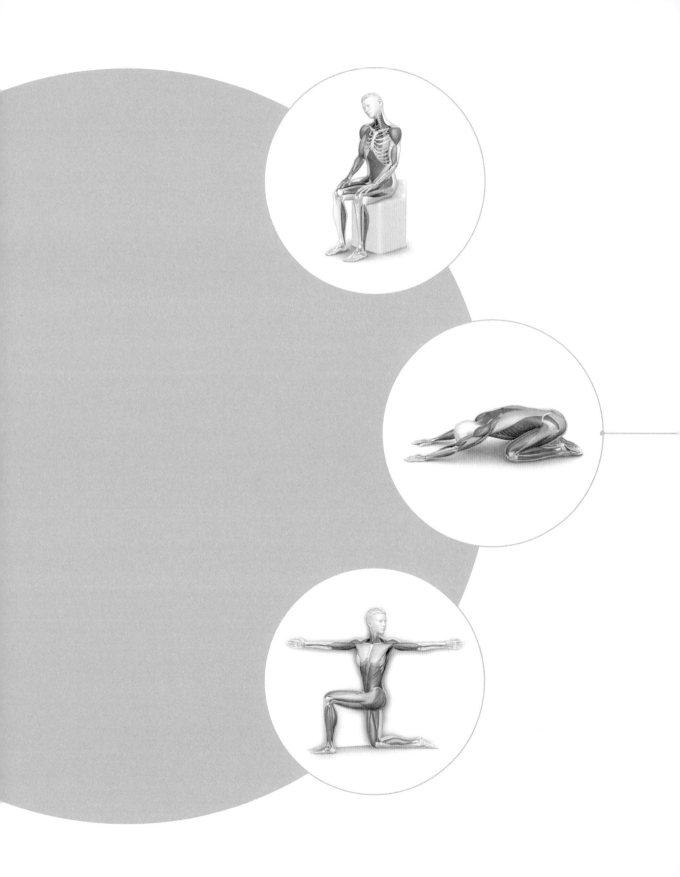

NECK AND SPINE EXERCISES

The spine is a hardworking part of the body. It allows for multiplanar movement of the trunk – forward and back, from side to side, and twisting right and left. It also supports the body and respiratory function, and protects the spinal cord and nerves. The neck, or cervical region of the spine, is the most mobile region and can become painful with overuse. These exercises encourage mobility in all parts of the spine, which can help reduce pain and stiffness and improve function.

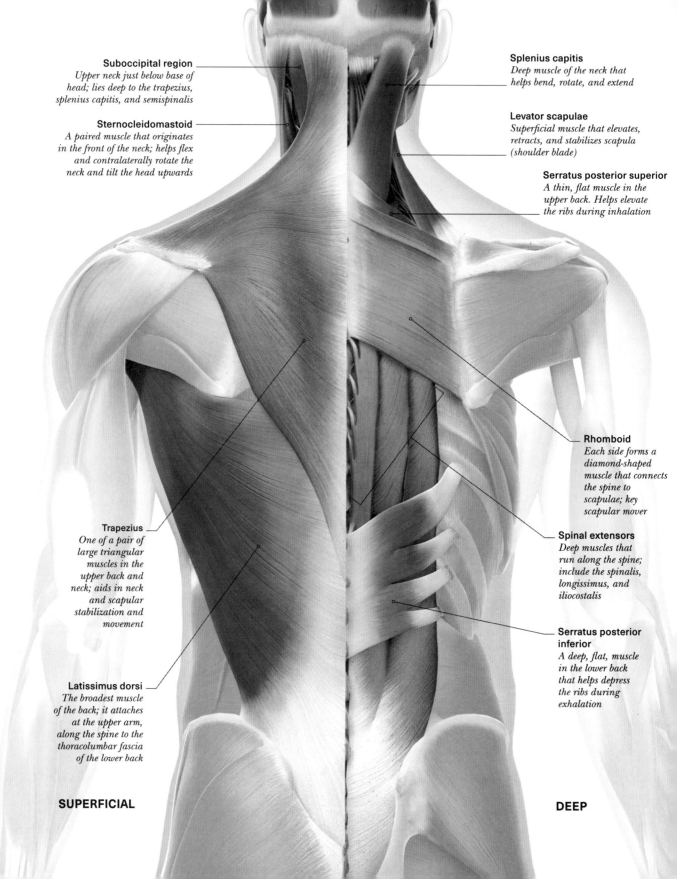

Suboccipital region
Upper neck just below base of head; lies deep to the trapezius, splenius capitis, and semispinalis

Sternocleidomastoid
A paired muscle that originates in the front of the neck; helps flex and contralaterally rotate the neck and tilt the head upwards

Splenius capitis
Deep muscle of the neck that helps bend, rotate, and extend

Levator scapulae
Superficial muscle that elevates, retracts, and stabilizes scapula (shoulder blade)

Serratus posterior superior
A thin, flat muscle in the upper back. Helps elevate the ribs during inhalation

Rhomboid
Each side forms a diamond-shaped muscle that connects the spine to scapulae; key scapular mover

Spinal extensors
Deep muscles that run along the spine; include the spinalis, longissimus, and iliocostalis

Trapezius
One of a pair of large triangular muscles in the upper back and neck; aids in neck and scapular stabilization and movement

Serratus posterior inferior
A deep, flat, muscle in the lower back that helps depress the ribs during exhalation

Latissimus dorsi
The broadest muscle of the back; it attaches at the upper arm, along the spine to the thoracolumbar fascia of the lower back

SUPERFICIAL

DEEP

NECK AND SPINE OVERVIEW

The major muscles of the neck and back include the trapezius, rhomboids, erector spinae, latissimus dorsi (lats), and the muscles of the cervical spine, such as the deep flexors, splenius, sternocleidomastoid, and scalene muscles. These muscles are crucial for maintaining posture and trunk stability, and moving the neck.

The neck and back muscles have important functions in supporting the head, in posture, and in facilitating movement in multiple planes. They also help with breathing. The trapezius and rhomboids are major scapular movers, aiding in shoulder movement and stability. The lats can adduct and extend the shoulder and are important muscles in rowing, swimming, and climbing. The spinal extensors extend the back and contribute to postural stability in everyday activities like sitting upright, carrying objects, and looking around you.

Stretching and strength training can reduce tension, and improve range of motion, strength, and endurance. Strength exercises to train this group include rows and pulldowns.

LEVATOR STRETCH

The neck is an area of the body that can hold tension for a variety of reasons: increased time spent with the shoulders elevated can contribute to tension, such as when sitting at a desk for long periods. Targeting the muscles that elevate the shoulders can help.

The levator scapulae muscle is located each side of the neck and attaches from the medial shoulder blade to the base of the skull. Use the Levator Stretch as part of a neck and shoulder exercise programme or as a stretch as needed.

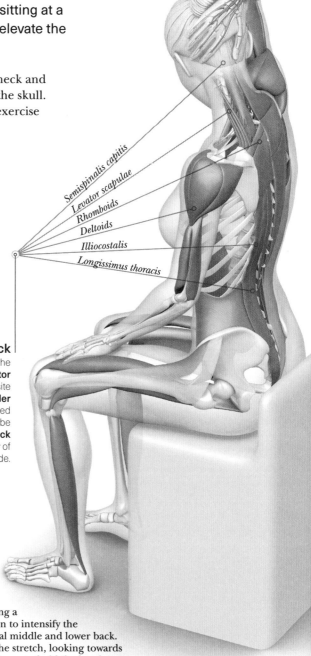

Semispinalis capitis
Levator scapulae
Rhomboids
Deltoids
Illiocostalis
Longissimus thoracis

KEY

- •-- *Joints*
- ○— *Muscles*
- ● Shortening with tension
- ● Lengthening with tension
- ● Lengthening without tension
- ● Held muscles without motion

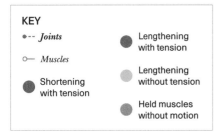

Look straight ahead with a relaxed neck

Keep your core neutral

Position legs hip-width apart, feet flat on floor

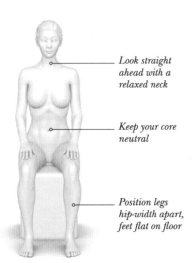

Arms and neck
Your right arm facilitates the stretch along the **levator scapulae** down the opposite side of the neck and **shoulder blade** with the sternum aimed forward. The stretch can be felt from the **posterior neck** down to the **medial border** of the shoulder blade.

PREPARATORY STAGE
Sit on a chair with shoulders relaxed and feet flat on the floor. Keep your gaze forward and spine neutral, hands resting lightly on your thighs.

STAGE ONE/TWO
Turn your head and neck to the right and down slightly, looking towards your right armpit. Place the palm of your right hand on the back of the head, using a downward arching motion to intensify the stretch. Maintain a neutral middle and lower back. Switch sides and repeat the stretch, looking towards the left and using the left arm to hold the head.

MANUAL SUBOCCIPITAL STRETCH

This gentle exercise can help reduce neck tension that originates in the four suboccipital muscles located at the base of the skull – the muscles responsible for tilting the head and chin upwards. The chin retraction and tuck (upper cervical flexion) in the stretch targets these.

This stretch may help relieve symptoms related to temporomandibular joint pain – the joints that connect your lower jaw to your skull – neck pain, or tension headaches. It can be used as part of a neck or jaw programme or simply as a stretch when needed, especially for those who work regularly on a computer.

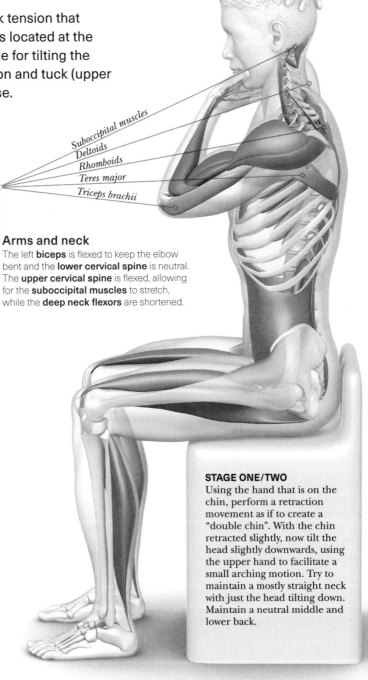

Suboccipital muscles
Deltoids
Rhomboids
Teres major
Triceps brachii

Arms and neck

The left **biceps** is flexed to keep the elbow bent and the **lower cervical spine** is neutral. The **upper cervical spine** is flexed, allowing for the **suboccipital muscles** to stretch, while the **deep neck flexors** are shortened.

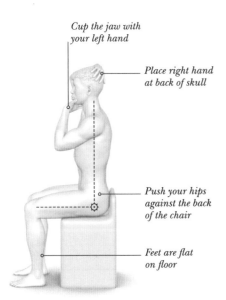

Cup the jaw with your left hand

Place right hand at back of skull

Push your hips against the back of the chair

Feet are flat on floor

PREPARATORY STAGE

Begin seated with feet flat on the floor, your gaze forward and spine neutral. Cup the chin with the left hand, using the webbing between the thumb and index finger. Place the right hand at the back of the skull.

STAGE ONE/TWO

Using the hand that is on the chin, perform a retraction movement as if to create a "double chin". With the chin retracted slightly, now tilt the head slightly downwards, using the upper hand to facilitate a small arching motion. Try to maintain a mostly straight neck with just the head tilting down. Maintain a neutral middle and lower back.

STERNOCLEIDOMASTOID (SCM) STRETCH

The SCM is a two-headed muscle that originates from the clavicle and attaches near the jaw. It is responsible for tilting the head up and drawing the neck forward. It can hold tension with sustained neck positions or laboured breathing habits.

This stretch may help relieve symptoms of tempromandibular pain (around the jaw), neck pain, or tension headaches. It can be used as part of a neck, jaw, and shoulder programme or as a stretch when needed. You may modify this by only doing the stage 1 part of the stretch if you feel this is enough; it should feel like a comfortable movement. Make sure you stay within a pain-free range of motion throughout the stretch.

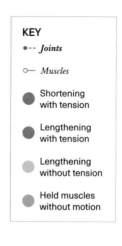

KEY

- •-- *Joints*
- o— *Muscles*
- Shortening with tension
- Lengthening with tension
- Lengthening without tension
- Held muscles without motion

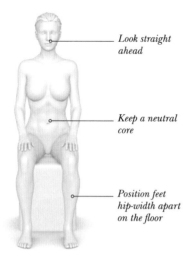

Look straight ahead

Keep a neutral core

Position feet hip-width apart on the floor

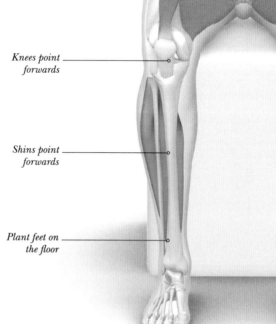

Knees point forwards

Shins point forwards

Plant feet on the floor

PREPARATORY STAGE
Begin seated with shoulders relaxed and feet flat on the floor, with your gaze forward and spine neutral.

66 99

The sternocleidomastoid muscle has two heads that can function individually or together.

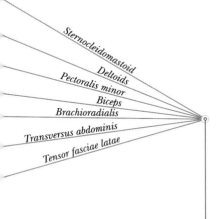

Sternocleidomastoid
Deltoids
Pectoralis minor
Biceps
Brachioradialis
Transversus abdominis
Tensor fasciae latae

Gaze is up and slightly to the right side

Overlap hands on clavicle of target side

Keep right shoulder relaxed

Maintain a neutral spine

Bend the right arm at the elbow

Keep hips level against back of the chair

Legs remain static

Trunk

As your head tilts back, The **sternocleidomastoid muscle** is lengthened. Your **hands** provide a counter stretch near the **sternal head**.

STAGE ONE
Place your right hand on your left clavicle, anchoring that hand with the left hand. Begin by tilting the chin upwards towards the ceiling. Maintain a relaxed breath.

STAGE TWO
Keeping the chin tilted upwards and neck slightly extended, bend the head and neck to the right. Maintain a neutral middle and lower back. Return to the preparatory stage, then complete the stretch on the other side.

71

SCALENE STRETCH

The three scalene muscles are located deep to the sternocleidomastoid muscle, and lateral to the cervical spine, attaching the vertebrae to the first two ribs. They assist with breathing, working as accessory breathing muscles to elevate the ribs. They also assist head and neck movement.

Increased tension or dysfunction in the scalene muscles can contribute to a variety of issues. These include neck pain, thoracic outlet syndrome (compression of nerves, arteries, and veins in the neck and chest), and decreased breathing capacity. The Scalene Stretch can be used as part of a neck and shoulder exercise programme or as a simple stretch as needed. You may modify the stretch by only performing the stage 1 level. Due to nerves and other structures in this area, it's important to stay within a comfortable range.

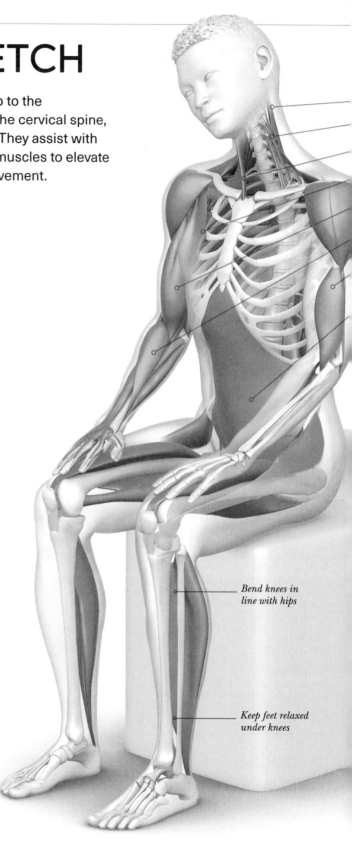

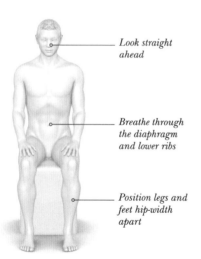

Look straight ahead

Breathe through the diaphragm and lower ribs

Position legs and feet hip-width apart

PREPARATORY STAGE
Sit on a chair with your shoulders relaxed and feet flat on the floor. Keep your gaze forward and spine neutral.

Bend knees in line with hips

Keep feet relaxed under knees

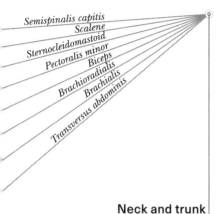

Semispinalis capitis
Scalene
Sternocleidomastoid
Pectoralis minor
Biceps
Brachioradialis
Brachialis
Transversus abdominis

Neck and trunk
The right **sternocleidomastoid muscle** laterally flexes the neck and the **intercostals** depress the **ribs** upon exhale to help facilitate a stretch in the **scalenes**.

" "

The brachial plexus, subclavian artery, subclavian vein, and phrenic nerve are all structures that pass through the scalenes at various points.

KEY

- •-- *Joints*
- ○— *Muscles*
- ● Shortening with tension
- ● Lengthening with tension
- ● Lengthening without tension
- ● Held muscles without motion

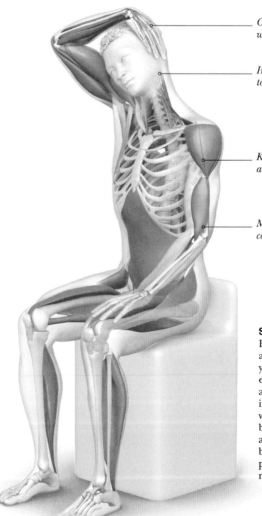

Cradle your left ear with your right hand

Intensify neck stretch to the right slightly

Keep your right arm relaxed

Maintain a neutral core and lower back

STAGE ONE
Begin by flexing the head and neck to the right. Maintain a relaxed breath, and keep your eye gaze forwards.

STAGE TWO
Bring your right arm up and cradle the head with your hand over the left ear. Use a sideways arching motion to intensify the stretch, without forcing the neck beyond comfort. Maintain a neutral core and low back. Return to the preparatory position and repeat on the other side.

73

CAT COW

The Cat pose mimics the position of a frightened cat; the Cow pose takes its name from the slight dip in the back typical of cows. Performed together in a flowing sequence as Cat Cow, this is a great stretch to enhance spinal mobility.

The movement of spinal flexion and spinal extension in Cat Cow mobilizes the spine and engages the abdominal and chest muscles. It's a perfect exercise to help reduce joint stiffness and can be used as a warmup or a daily routine.

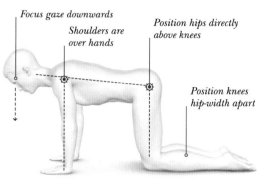

Focus gaze downwards

Shoulders are over hands

Position hips directly above knees

Position knees hip-width apart

PREPARATORY STAGE
Begin in four-point kneeling position with the shoulders above the wrists, the hips above the knees, and the head and neck in line. Keep your spine neutral: this refers to your middle, comfortable zone between fully flexed and fully extended.

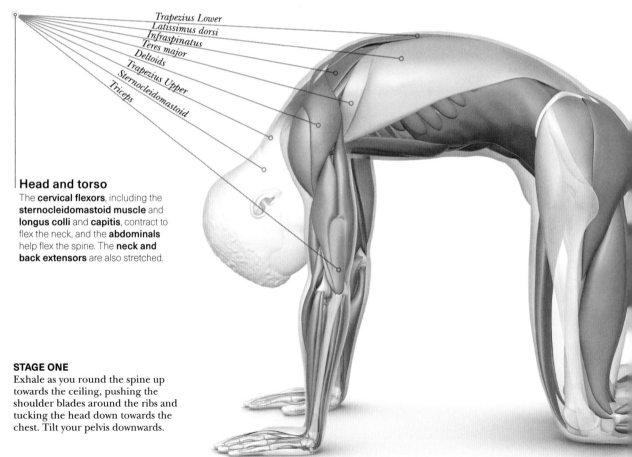

Trapezius Lower
Latissimus dorsi
Infraspinatus
Teres major
Deltoids
Trapezius Upper
Sternocleidomastoid
Triceps

Head and torso
The **cervical flexors**, including the **sternocleidomastoid muscle** and **longus colli** and **capitis**, contract to flex the neck, and the **abdominals** help flex the spine. The **neck and back extensors** are also stretched.

STAGE ONE
Exhale as you round the spine up towards the ceiling, pushing the shoulder blades around the ribs and tucking the head down towards the chest. Tilt your pelvis downwards.

KEY

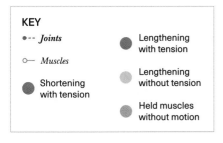

- •-- *Joints*
- ○— *Muscles*
- ● Shortening with tension
- ● Lengthening with tension
- ● Lengthening without tension
- ● Held muscles without motion

VARIATION: SEATED

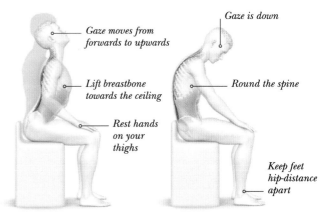

Gaze moves from forwards to upwards

Lift breastbone towards the ceiling

Rest hands on your thighs

Gaze is down

Round the spine

Keep feet hip-distance apart

PREP / STAGE ONE   STAGE TWO

PREPARATORY STAGE
Sit tall on a chair with hands resting on your thighs and feet flat on the floor. Assume a neutral spine where you feel most upright and comfortable.

STAGE ONE
Begin by inhaling and letting the spine arch as you look upwards, simultaneously lifting your breastbone towards the ceiling. Attempt to extend and move through the whole spine in one fluid motion.

STAGE TWO
Exhale and round the spine downwards so that the head tilts down and the breastbone is directed towards your hips. Tilt your head and neck downwards towards the chest at the same time.

Raise your head and look straight ahead

Squeeze shoulder blades towards the centre

Press the floor with your palms

Keep knees hip-distance apart

STAGE TWO
Inhale and let your belly sink towards the floor, raising your head and neck and curving your spine downwards simultaneously. Attempt to extend and move through the whole spine in one fluid motion.

QUADRATUS LUMBORUM (QL) STRETCH

The quadratus lumborum, located in the posterior abdominal wall, is the deepest back muscle. It contributes to stabilization of the lumbar spine and lateral bending, and is also an accessory breathing muscle. Overusing the QL can cause back pain.

The QL Stretch can help reduce back and shoulder tension or tightness along the outside of the hip. By crossing over one leg and reaching overhead, you can stretch the lateral muscles of the body from the shoulder to below the pelvis. Use this stretch as part of a hip, back, or shoulder programme, or simply as needed.

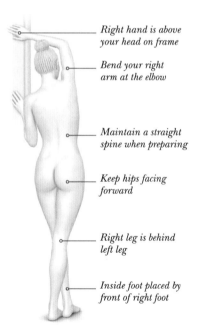

Right hand is above your head on frame

Bend your right arm at the elbow

Maintain a straight spine when preparing

Keep hips facing forward

Right leg is behind left leg

Inside foot placed by front of right foot

PREPARATORY STAGE
Begin standing in front of a doorway with the left leg crossed over the right leg. Place the right arm above your head on the doorframe, and the left arm in front of you against the frame, elbow bent. Stand upright and look straight ahead.

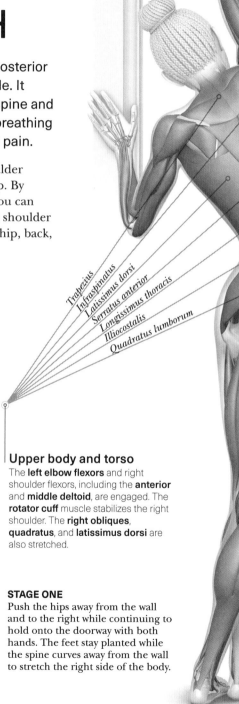

Trapezius
Infraspinatus
Latissimus dorsi
Serratus anterior
Longissimus thoracis
Illiocostalis
Quadratus lumborum

Upper body and torso
The **left elbow flexors** and right shoulder flexors, including the **anterior** and **middle deltoid**, are engaged. The **rotator cuff** muscle stabilizes the right shoulder. The **right obliques**, **quadratus**, and **latissimus dorsi** are also stretched.

STAGE ONE
Push the hips away from the wall and to the right while continuing to hold onto the doorway with both hands. The feet stay planted while the spine curves away from the wall to stretch the right side of the body.

KEY

- • - - *Joints*
- ○ - *Muscles*
- ● Shortening with tension
- ● Lengthening with tension
- ○ Lengthening without tension
- ● Held muscles without motion

Keep your trunk neutral during the stretch

Lower body

The **right gastrocnemius** is stretched, while the **hamstrings** and **glutes** engage to stabilize the hip. The **posterior tibialis**, **peroneals**, and **flexor hallucis longus** work to stabilize the left foot and ankle.

Gluteus medius
Vastus lateralis
Adductor magnus
Semitendinosus
mimembranosus
Biceps femoris
Gastrocnemius

Legs return to straight in stage 2 position

Feet are planted firmly on floor

VARIATION: SEATED

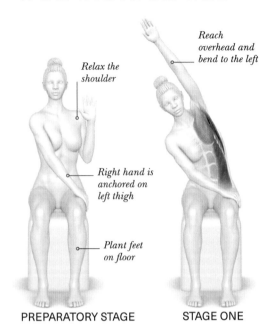

Relax the shoulder

Reach overhead and bend to the left

Right hand is anchored on left thigh

Plant feet on floor

PREPARATORY STAGE

STAGE ONE

PREPARATORY STAGE
Begin sitting with feet on the floor, with a neutral spine and your gaze forward. Place your right hand on the outside of your left thigh and hold your left hand up at about shoulder height.

STAGE ONE
Reach the left arm overhead and in an arching motion to the right, while keeping the right hand on the left thigh. Exhale as you move overhead. The spine should bend to the right as you reach.

STAGE TWO
Return to the preparatory stage by bringing the left arm back down to about shoulder height and straightening the spine.

STAGE TWO
Bring the hips back towards the door to achieve a straight spine once again. Return the arms to the preparatory position, with your gaze forward and an upright stance.

77

CHILD'S POSE

This restorative stretch relaxes the back and pelvis and stretches out the arms and ankles. The gentle spinal flexion can help with tension relief, especially around the lower back. It can also reduce joint stiffness.

Add a lateral variation (see right) to target the sides of the back and the latissimus dorsi muscles. Stay within a comfortable range and don't push your limits. Relax into the stretch by using your breath.

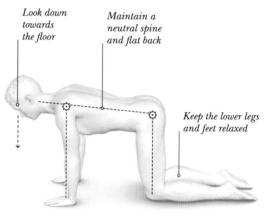

Look down towards the floor

Maintain a neutral spine and flat back

Keep the lower legs and feet relaxed

Neck and arms
Your **splenius capitis** and **splenius cervicus** neck muscles stretch, as well as your **posterior deltoids**. Your **arm muscles** serve as an anchor on the reach, stretching the shoulders overhead.

PREPARATORY STAGE
Begin in four-point kneeling with your shoulders above your wrists, hips above your knees, and your head and neck in line. Keep your spine neutral – in the middle, comfortable zone between fully flexed and fully extended.

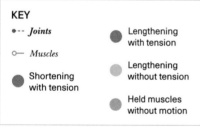

KEY

- ● -- *Joints*
- ○— *Muscles*
- ● Shortening with tension
- ● Lengthening with tension
- ● Lengthening without tension
- ● Held muscles without motion

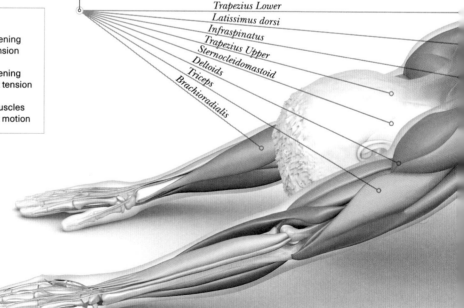

Trapezius Lower
Latissimus dorsi
Infraspinatus
Trapezius Upper
Sternocleidomastoid
Deltoids
Triceps
Brachioradialis

STAGE ONE
Slowly sit back on your heels and stretch your arms out in front of you, palms on the floor. Let your torso sink between your legs in a fold, and relax your back and shoulders as you exhale.

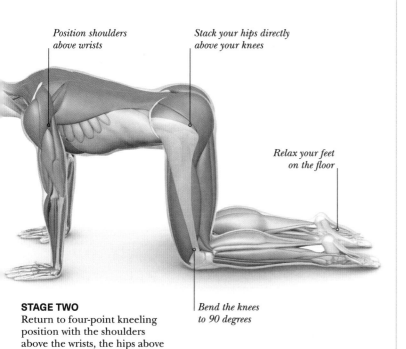

Position shoulders above wrists

Stack your hips directly above your knees

Relax your feet on the floor

Bend the knees to 90 degrees

STAGE TWO
Return to four-point kneeling position with the shoulders above the wrists, the hips above the knees, and the head and neck in line.

VARIATION: LATERAL POSE

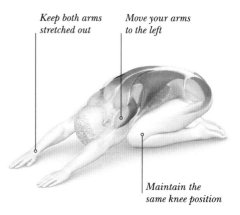

Keep both arms stretched out

Move your arms to the left

Maintain the same knee position

ALTERNATIVE STAGE TWO
Walk hands to one side of the body, keeping them stretched out in front of you. Repeat to the other side.

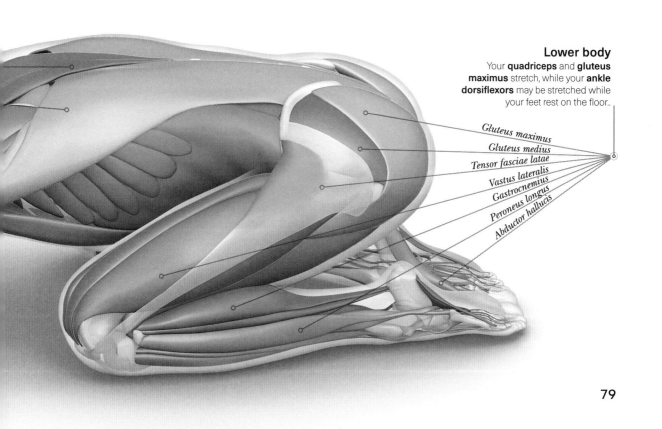

Lower body
Your **quadriceps** and **gluteus maximus** stretch, while your **ankle dorsiflexors** may be stretched while your feet rest on the floor..

Gluteus maximus
Gluteus medius
Tensor fasciae latae
Vastus lateralis
Gastrocnemius
Peroneus longus
Abductor hallucis

COBRA

The Cobra is a popular yoga position that helps to stretch the abdominals and hip flexors, and promotes mobility into spinal extension. It can be used as part of a daily stretch routine, or if you want to improve the flexibility of your spine.

While your chest extends and your abdominals and hips are placed on stretch, the muscles in your back, shoulders, and arms activate to hold the pose. Be mindful of any discomfort or pain in the back or shoulders, and make modifications as necessary, such as not pushing up too high, until you get used to the stretch.

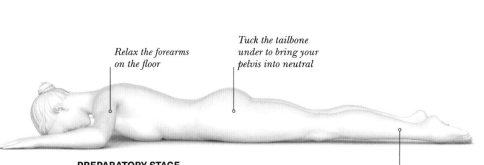

Relax the forearms on the floor

Tuck the tailbone under to bring your pelvis into neutral

Legs and feet rotate outwards

PREPARATORY STAGE
Lie face-down on the floor with your legs slightly wider than hip-width apart. Rest your forehead on the floor, lengthening your neck and tucking the chin slightly. Place your arms out to the sides with your elbows bent to 90 degrees, your forearms flat on the floor, and your palms downwards. Inhale, and gently tuck your tailbone under to begin.

KEY

●--- *Joints*

○— *Muscles*

● Shortening with tension

● Lengthening with tension

● Lengthening without tension

● Held muscles without motion

Upper body

The **neck extensors** keep the head lifted upright; the **spinal extensors** activate to extend your spine. Your **abdominal muscles** lengthen and your **periscapular muscles** engage to draw your scapulae together.

Sternocleidomastoid
Semispinalis capitis
Deltoids
Teres major
Serratus anterior
External oblique
Quadratus lumborum
Internal oblique

VARIATION: TWISTED COBRA

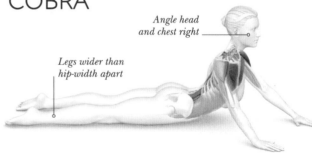

Angle head and chest right

Legs wider than hip-width apart

STAGE ONE

In the full Cobra position, gently walk both hands towards the right side, keeping the elbows extended. Maintain a long trunk and try not to collapse down on one side. Keep your chest lifted and collar bones wide. Inhale to hold the position, and then exhale as you walk the hands over to the left side to repeat.

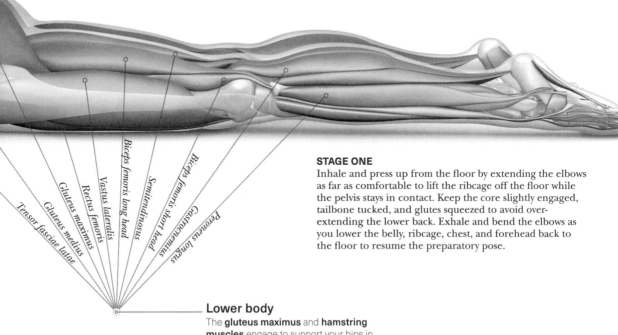

Biceps femoris long head
Biceps femoris short head
Semitendinosus
Gastrocnemius
Vastus lateralis
Peroneus longus
Rectus femoris
Gluteus maximus
Gluteus medius
Tensor fasciae latae

STAGE ONE

Inhale and press up from the floor by extending the elbows as far as comfortable to lift the ribcage off the floor while the pelvis stays in contact. Keep the core slightly engaged, tailbone tucked, and glutes squeezed to avoid over-extending the lower back. Exhale and bend the elbows as you lower the belly, ribcage, chest, and forehead back to the floor to resume the preparatory pose.

Lower body

The **gluteus maximus** and **hamstring muscles** engage to support your hips in the pose. The **hip flexors** lengthen. Your **gluteus medius** and **minimus** help to with stabilize your hips. Your **quadriceps** in the front of the thighs engage to support knee extension.

» VARIATIONS

These two variations for the Cobra pose put less pressure on the shoulder and create less of an angle for the lower back. They are suitable for those who have wrist or shoulder limitations and can't press up, but still would like to achieve a spinal extension stretch.

HANDS FAR AWAY

Placing the hands further away means there is less extension in the lumbar spine. This modification is a more suitable option for those who are sensitive to, or have limitations in, extension of the spine. You may also start here and progress into more extension by bringing the hands closer to the sides in order to press up further.

KEY

● Primary target muscle

● Secondary target muscle

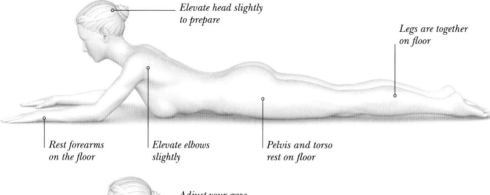

Elevate head slightly
to prepare

Legs are together
on floor

Rest forearms
on the floor

Elevate elbows
slightly

Pelvis and torso
rest on floor

PREPARATORY STAGE
Begin lying on your front with elbows slightly bent and arms out in front.

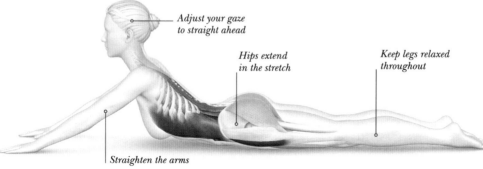

Adjust your gaze
to straight ahead

Hips extend
in the stretch

Keep legs relaxed
throughout

Straighten the arms

STAGE ONE
Exhale to push up from the floor with the forearms by pressing the elbows to extend the chest up. Keep the core slightly engaged, tailbone tucked, and glutes squeezed. Lift the belly slightly off the floor.

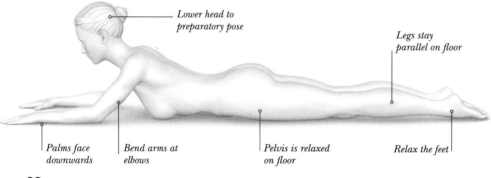

Lower head to
preparatory pose

Legs stay
parallel on floor

Palms face
downwards

Bend arms at
elbows

Pelvis is relaxed
on floor

Relax the feet

STAGE TWO
Slowly lower down, returning your gaze to the floor.

Stretches and exercises can be modified for individual abilities, which may vary at any given time.

ON ELBOWS

This modification for the Cobra pose puts less pressure on the shoulder and hands and less extension in the lower back. It's helpful for those who have wrist or shoulder limitations and can't press up but still would like to achieve a spinal extension stretch. It can be used as part of a daily stretch routine or to address mobility in the spine.

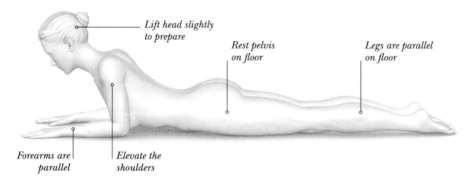

Lift head slightly to prepare

Rest pelvis on floor

Legs are parallel on floor

Forearms are parallel

Elevate the shoulders

PREPARATORY STAGE
Begin lying prone on the floor with elbows bent and forearms parallel.

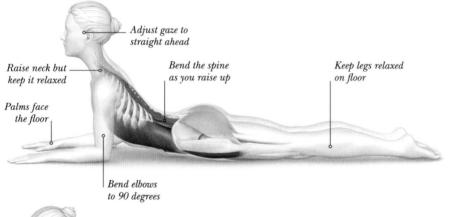

Adjust gaze to straight ahead

Raise neck but keep it relaxed

Bend the spine as you raise up

Keep legs relaxed on floor

Palms face the floor

Bend elbows to 90 degrees

STAGE ONE
Exhale to push up from the floor with the forearms by pressing the elbows to extend the chest up while exhaling. Engage the core slightly, tuck your tailbone, and squeeze your glutes to avoid over-extending the lower back, then lift the belly off the floor.

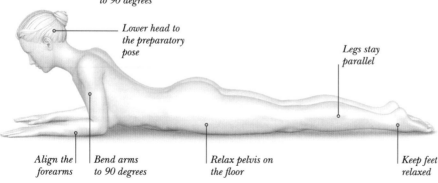

Lower head to the preparatory pose

Legs stay parallel

Align the forearms

Bend arms to 90 degrees

Relax pelvis on the floor

Keep feet relaxed

STAGE TWO
Slowly lower down, returning your gaze to the floor.

STANDING THORACIC EXTENSION WALL STRETCH

All you need is a wall to perform this simple stretch to help target upper back and shoulder stiffness. It can be used as part of a daily stretch routine or to address mobility in the spine, neck pain, and shoulder range of motion.

Thoracic mobility can influence shoulder range of motion and posture, particularly in the middle and lower back region. Keeping this area mobile can be extremely beneficial for healthy upper body function. The Standing

Thoracic Extension Wall Stretch elongates the upper back and is often prescribed to those with neck, shoulder, or upper back pain. You can customize how far you spread your fingers apart to what feels most comfortable for you.

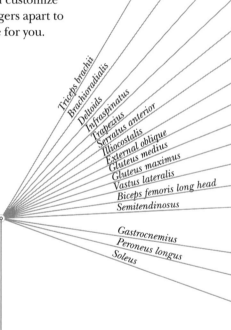

Triceps brachii
Brachioradialis
Deltoids
Infraspinatus
Trapezius
Serratus anterior
Illiocostalis
External oblique
Gluteus medius
Gluteus maximus
Vastus lateralis
Biceps femoris long head
Semitendinosus

Gastrocnemius
Peroneus longus
Soleus

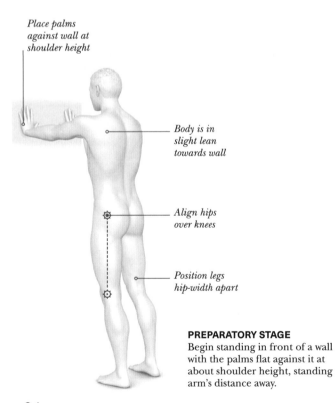

Place palms against wall at shoulder height

Body is in slight lean towards wall

Align hips over knees

Position legs hip-width apart

PREPARATORY STAGE
Begin standing in front of a wall with the palms flat against it at about shoulder height, standing arm's distance away.

Upper and lower body
The **triceps** stabilize the elbows and the **serratus anterior** and **pectoral muscles** help stabilize the shoulders as they're flexed. The **latissimus dorsi** and **subscapularis** are also stretched. The **spinal extensors** extend the thoracic spine. The **hip flexors** and **quads** engage to flex the hips and stabilize the knees so that the **hamstrings** are stretched.

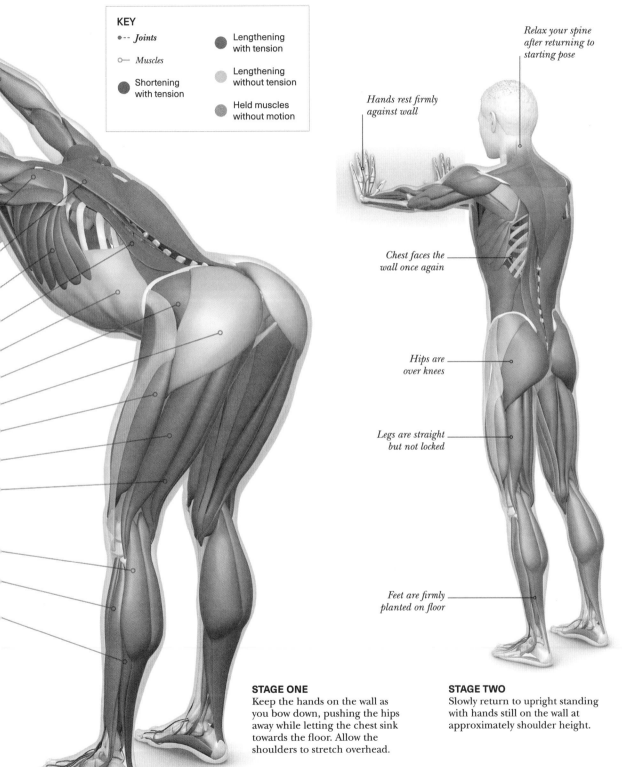

KEY

- • -- *Joints*
- ○— *Muscles*
- ● Shortening with tension
- ● Lengthening with tension
- ○ Lengthening without tension
- ◐ Held muscles without motion

Relax your spine after returning to starting pose

Hands rest firmly against wall

Chest faces the wall once again

Hips are over knees

Legs are straight but not locked

Feet are firmly planted on floor

STAGE ONE
Keep the hands on the wall as you bow down, pushing the hips away while letting the chest sink towards the floor. Allow the shoulders to stretch overhead.

STAGE TWO
Slowly return to upright standing with hands still on the wall at approximately shoulder height.

» VARIATIONS

These variations can be done on the floor, which involves less hamstring engagement compared to standing. They may be more demanding on the arms, but can offer a more intense thoracic extension stretch.

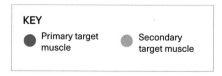

KEY

● Primary target muscle   ● Secondary target muscle

ARMS ON A CHAIR

This variation is a great way to intensify the stretch by bending the elbows and extending through a shorter distance. The exercise addresses thoracic mobility, shoulder mobility, and latissimus dorsi (lat) flexibility, and can be used to relieve pain or stiffness in the neck and shoulder.

PREPARATORY STAGE
Begin kneeling with your elbows resting on a chair and hands relaxed on your upper back, the upper back flexed over the chair.

STAGE ONE
Slowly extend through the upper back and sit back towards your heels. Let the neck and thoracic spine extend naturally.

STAGE TWO
Push yourself back up to the preparatory position to come out of the stretch.

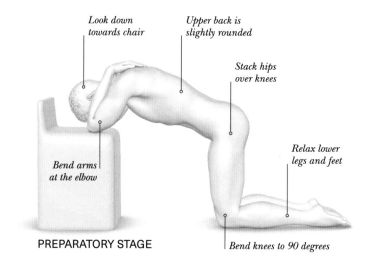

Look down towards chair

Upper back is slightly rounded

Stack hips over knees

Bend arms at the elbow

Relax lower legs and feet

Bend knees to 90 degrees

PREPARATORY STAGE

PUPPY POSE

The Puppy Pose is a yoga pose that encourages the same thoracic extension as the main stretch, but with the arms extended and the use of the floor. It is a great stretch for relaxation, and can be used as part of a daily stretch routine or to address mobility issues in the hips.

PREPARATORY STAGE
Begin on all fours on the floor with arms slightly in front of your shoulders.

STAGE ONE
Walk the hands further forward and let the chest lower to the floor while keeping the hips high and the knees bent.

STAGE TWO
Return to the preparatory position.

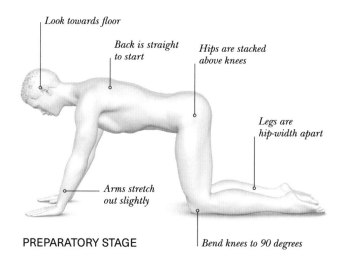

Look towards floor

Back is straight to start

Hips are stacked above knees

Legs are hip-width apart

Arms stretch out slightly

Bend knees to 90 degrees

PREPARATORY STAGE

66 99

Varying hand and shoulder positioning changes where a stretch will target most.

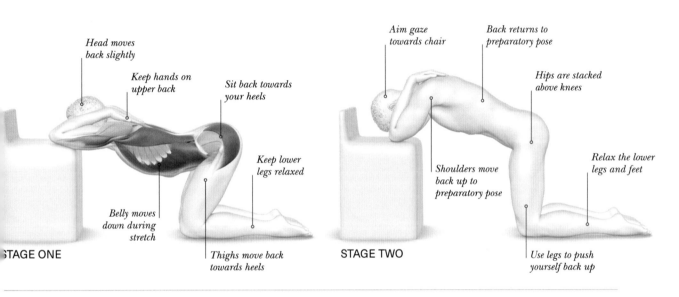

STAGE ONE

Head moves back slightly

Keep hands on upper back

Sit back towards your heels

Keep lower legs relaxed

Belly moves down during stretch

Thighs move back towards heels

STAGE TWO

Aim gaze towards chair

Back returns to preparatory pose

Hips are stacked above knees

Shoulders move back up to preparatory pose

Relax the lower legs and feet

Use legs to push yourself back up

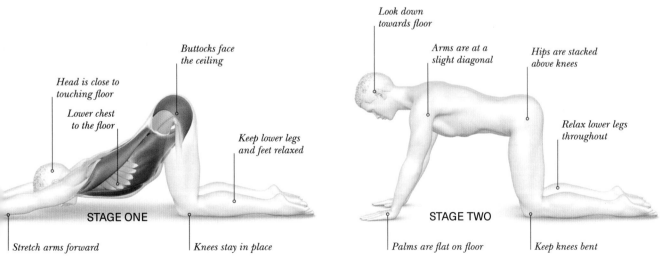

STAGE ONE

Buttocks face the ceiling

Head is close to touching floor

Lower chest to the floor

Keep lower legs and feet relaxed

Stretch arms forward

Knees stay in place

STAGE TWO

Look down towards floor

Arms are at a slight diagonal

Hips are stacked above knees

Relax lower legs throughout

Palms are flat on floor

Keep knees bent

HALF-KNEEL THORACIC ROTATION

Rotation of the thorax (between the neck and diaphragm), motor control, and strength are required for multiplanar activity – when you move your body up and down, from side to side, and forwards and backwards. Regularly addressing mobility in the thorax may reduce excessive load or stress in neighboring regions, like the shoulder or neck. This chest-opening movement is an excellent exercise to target these regions.

This is a great stretch for any multidirectional athlete, especially those who play basketball, tennis, golf, and football. The half-kneel position, against a wall, prevents your lumbar (lower back) region from moving to compensate. It is often prescribed for back, neck, or shoulder pain.

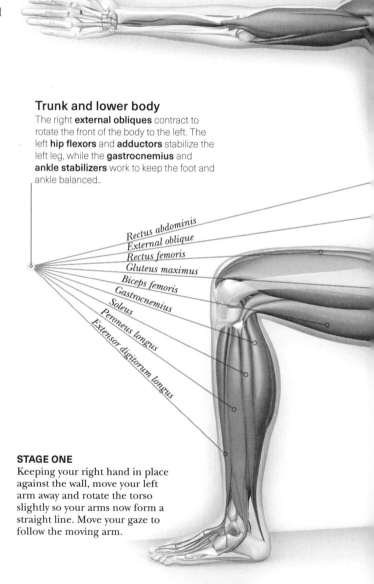

Trunk and lower body
The right **external obliques** contract to rotate the front of the body to the left. The left **hip flexors** and **adductors** stabilize the left leg, while the **gastrocnemius** and **ankle stabilizers** work to keep the foot and ankle balanced..

Rectus abdominis
External oblique
Rectus femoris
Gluteus maximus
Biceps femoris
Gastrocnemius
Soleus
Peroneus longus
Extensor digitorum longus

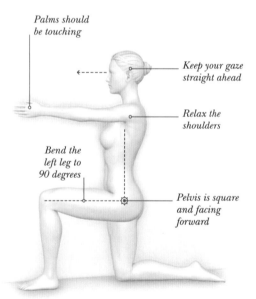

Palms should be touching

Keep your gaze straight ahead

Relax the shoulders

Bend the left leg to 90 degrees

Pelvis is square and facing forward

PREPARATORY STAGE
Begin in the half-kneel position, with your right knee on the floor next to a wall and the left knee in front, bent to 90 degrees. Stretch both arms out in front, palms touching each other and hips square. Rest your right hand against the wall.

STAGE ONE
Keeping your right hand in place against the wall, move your left arm away and rotate the torso slightly so your arms now form a straight line. Move your gaze to follow the moving arm.

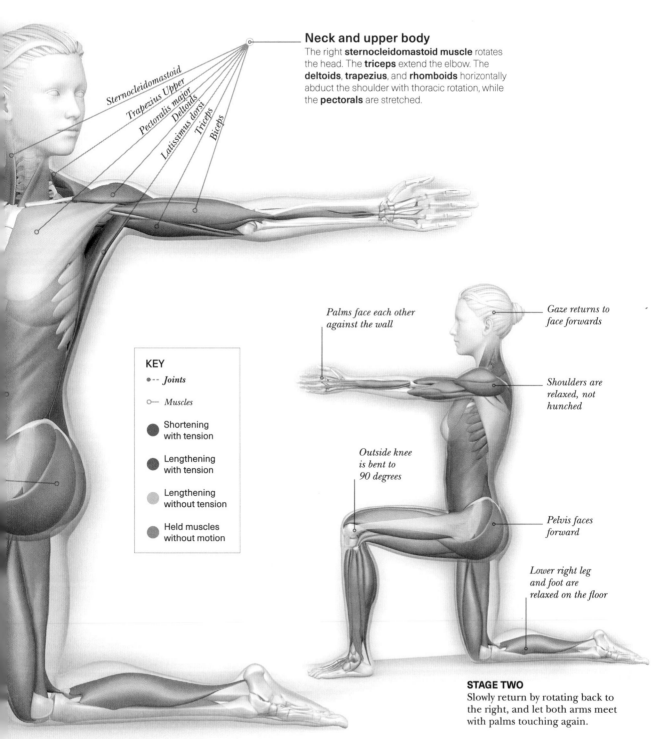

Neck and upper body

The right **sternocleidomastoid muscle** rotates the head. The **triceps** extend the elbow. The **deltoids**, **trapezius**, and **rhomboids** horizontally abduct the shoulder with thoracic rotation, while the **pectorals** are stretched.

Sternocleidomastoid

Trapezius Upper

Pectoralis major

Deltoids

Latissimus dorsi

Triceps

Biceps

KEY

●-- *Joints*

○— *Muscles*

● Shortening with tension

● Lengthening with tension

● Lengthening without tension

● Held muscles without motion

Palms face each other against the wall

Gaze returns to face forwards

Shoulders are relaxed, not hunched

Outside knee is bent to 90 degrees

Pelvis faces forward

Lower right leg and foot are relaxed on the floor

STAGE TWO

Slowly return by rotating back to the right, and let both arms meet with palms touching again.

89

» VARIATIONS

Depending on someone's ability to kneel or their available hip range of motion, the standing variation of the Half-Kneel Thoracic Rotation may be a more comfortable option for the lower body.

STANDING THORACIC ROTATION

You can easily add this variation to the start or end of a workout, or fit it in during a lunch break. Because your trunk is not fixed like it is when you are on the floor, your pelvis will move with you as you rotate.

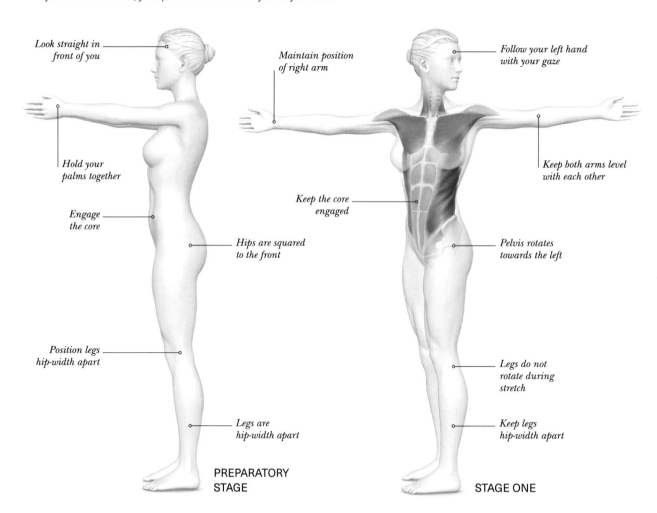

Look straight in front of you

Maintain position of right arm

Follow your left hand with your gaze

Hold your palms together

Keep the core engaged

Keep both arms level with each other

Engage the core

Hips are squared to the front

Pelvis rotates towards the left

Position legs hip-width apart

Legs do not rotate during stretch

Legs are hip-width apart

Keep legs hip-width apart

PREPARATORY STAGE

STAGE ONE

PREPARATORY STAGE
Stand tall with your feet hip-width apart and your spine and pelvis in neutral. Raise both arms up to shoulder height, with your shoulders relaxed and your palms facing each other.

STAGE ONE
Exhale to open your left arm out towards the left and behind you as far as you can, rotating your spine and head at the same time. Keep the right arm lengthened and still.

STAGE TWO
Inhale as you return back to the preparatory position. Repeat on the opposite side and continue alternating sides.

BRETZEL

The Bretzel stretch combines thoracic rotation in the sidelying position with the legs split to maintain the position of the pelvis. Additionally, the knee is pulled into flexion with the arm that is rotated away, allowing for a quad and pec stretch.

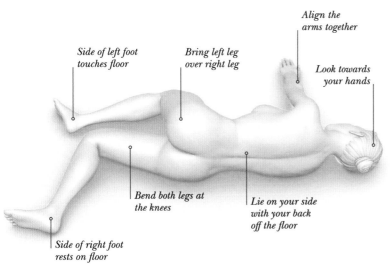

Side of left foot touches floor

Bring left leg over right leg

Align the arms together

Look towards your hands

Bend both legs at the knees

Lie on your side with your back off the floor

Side of right foot rests on floor

PREPARATORY STAGE

Begin lying on your right side with the legs relaxed and bent, the top leg crossed over the bottom one and resting on the floor. Extend the arms in front of you and place the palms together.

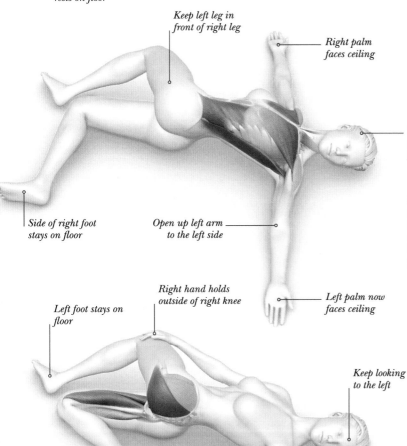

Keep left leg in front of right leg

Right palm faces ceiling

Twist head and neck to follow your left arm

Side of right foot stays on floor

Open up left arm to the left side

Right hand holds outside of right knee

Left palm now faces ceiling

Left foot stays on floor

Keep looking to the left

Grasp right foot with left hand

Left shoulder rests on floor

STAGE ONE

Open up the chest by rotating the upper body to the left left and resting the left arm on the floor, keeping position of the lower body in place. Follow the movement of your left arm with your gaze.

STAGE TWO

Place the right hand on top of the right knee and grasp the left foot with the left hand, bringing the lower body into a stretch.

STANDING HALF MOON

This thoracic rotation, performed against a wall, is an excellent exercise to target upper back rotation. It helps improve mobility in the spine, neck, and shoulder, and is perfect for a daily stretch routine.

The floor modification of the Half Moon rotation is a good alternative that is less vigorous for the rotating side. It's an excellent option for anyone who can't tolerate the standing version, such as those who experience back pain with rotation or difficulty holding their arms in the air.

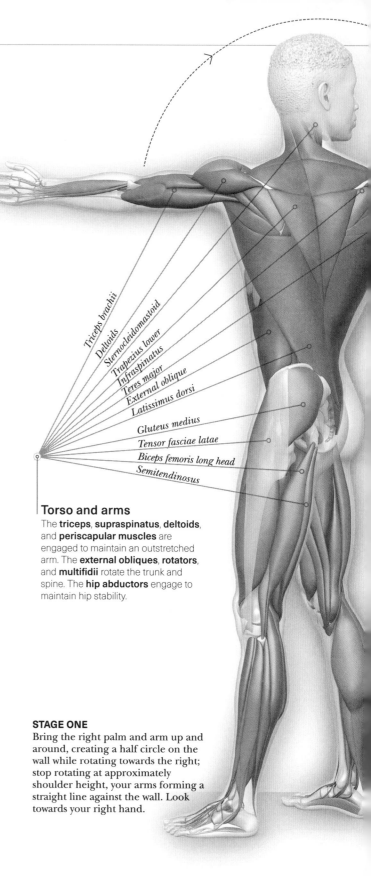

Triceps brachii
Deltoids
Sternocleidomastoid
Trapezius lower
Infraspinatus
Teres major
External oblique
Latissimus dorsi
Gluteus medius
Tensor fasciae latae
Biceps femoris long head
Semitendinosus

Torso and arms
The **triceps**, **supraspinatus**, **deltoids**, and **periscapular muscles** are engaged to maintain an outstretched arm. The **external obliques**, **rotators**, and **multifidii** rotate the trunk and spine. The **hip abductors** engage to maintain hip stability.

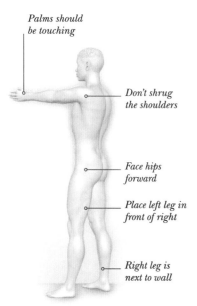

Palms should be touching

Don't shrug the shoulders

Face hips forward

Place left leg in front of right

Right leg is next to wall

PREPARATORY STAGE
Begin in a split stance next to a wall on your right with your left leg slightly in front of your right leg, arms stretched out in front. Place your palms against each other and keep your hips square, facing forward.

STAGE ONE
Bring the right palm and arm up and around, creating a half circle on the wall while rotating towards the right; stop rotating at approximately shoulder height, your arms forming a straight line against the wall. Look towards your right hand.

VARIATION: HALF MOON ON FLOOR

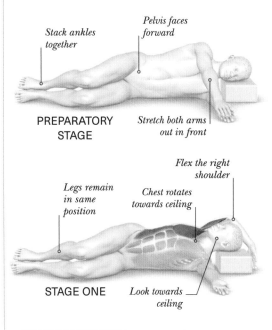

Stack ankles together

Pelvis faces forward

PREPARATORY STAGE

Stretch both arms out in front

Legs remain in same position

Flex the right shoulder

Chest rotates towards ceiling

STAGE ONE

Look towards ceiling

KEY

- •-- *Joints*
- ○— *Muscles*
- ● Shortening with tension
- ● Lengthening with tension
- ● Lengthening without tension
- ● Held muscles without motion

Focus your gaze forwards

Return right hand to original position

Maintain an upright posture

Right leg slightly back throughout movement

Left leg slightly in front of right

STAGE TWO

Return the right palm by creating the same half circle back and rotating the torso back to facing forward.

PREPARATORY STAGE

Lie on your left side with your head supported on a block and arms stretched out in front, palms facing each other and hips square. Flex your hips and knees.

STAGE ONE

Keeping the left arm stretched in front, bring the right palm and arm up to your chest, and then out to the right side, letting your spine and head rotate to the right to follow it.

STAGE TWO

Return the right hand by creating the same half circle back and rotating the torso back towards the front to stack the hands.

! Caution

Create a big motion with the moving arm to facilitate scapular motion. If you experience any discomfort or pain in the neck, back, or shoulders, make whatever modifications are needed, such as not moving as far into the stretch.

THREAD THE NEEDLE

This simple mobility exercise can help reduce stiffness and improve rotation in the thoracic spine. It also contributes to improved function and mobility in the neck and shoulder.

Thread the Needle includes the rotation of the upper back with one fixed arm serving as an anchor. It can be used as a warmup, daily stretch, or as part of a focussed upper body programme. It is commonly used as part of a greater mobility sequence for the upper body, and by those who play rotational sports such as tennis. It is also a popular exercise in yoga and Pilates classses.

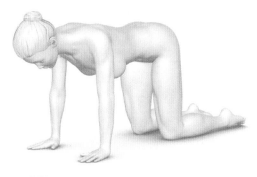

PREPARATORY STAGE
Begin in the four-point kneeling position with the shoulders stacked above the wrists, the hips above the knees, and the head and neck in line. Keep your spine and pelvis neutral.

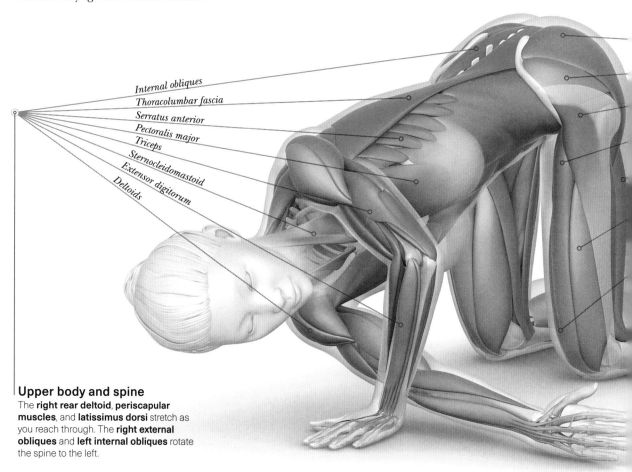

Internal obliques
Thoracolumbar fascia
Serratus anterior
Pectoralis major
Triceps
Sternocleidomastoid
Extensor digitorum
Deltoids

Upper body and spine
The **right rear deltoid, periscapular muscles**, and **latissimus dorsi** stretch as you reach through. The **right external obliques** and **left internal obliques** rotate the spine to the left.

Caution

Move with intention and control, following the reaching arm with the head and neck. Modify for wrist pain by placing a towel roll under the heels of the palms. If you experience knee pain, place a pad under the knees for comfort.

Lower body

The **gluteals** and **hip abductors** engage to stabilize the hips as the trunk lowers and rotates. The **toe extensors** and **ankle dorsiflexors** are stretched against the floor.

Gluteus maximus
Gluteus medius
Tensor fasciae latae
Rectus femoris
Biceps femoris long head
Vastus lateralis
Vastus medialis

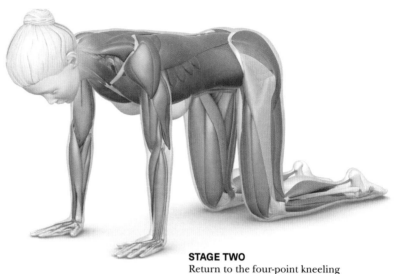

STAGE TWO
Return to the four-point kneeling position with the shoulders above the wrists, the hips above the knees, and the head and neck in line. You can add variety by reaching the right arm towards the ceiling for increased rotation in the opposite direction.

❝ ❞

The rotational element of Thread the Needle allows for thoracic mobility, an important region to address for shoulder and neck function.

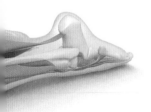

STAGE ONE
With your left hand fixed on the floor, reach through the space between the left arm and thighs and rotate through the thoracic spine.

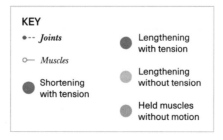

KEY

•-- *Joints*

○— *Muscles*

● Shortening with tension

● Lengthening with tension

● Lengthening without tension

● Held muscles without motion

≫ VARIATIONS

You can improve thoracic mobility by practising a variety of stretches that emphasize motion at this area of the spine. They can be very beneficial to help move you through different planes of motion.

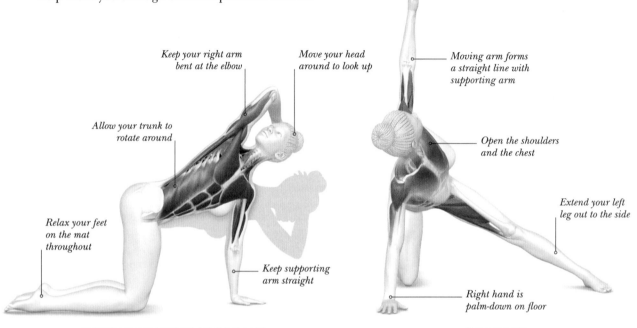

Keep your right arm bent at the elbow

Move your head around to look up

Moving arm forms a straight line with supporting arm

Allow your trunk to rotate around

Open the shoulders and the chest

Extend your left leg out to the side

Relax your feet on the mat throughout

Keep supporting arm straight

Right hand is palm-down on floor

PREPARATORY STAGE / STAGE ONE

STAGE ONE

HAND BEHIND HEAD

If you place your hand behind your head you reduce the arm lever length, which helps if you have tight or tender shoulders. You can then focus more on trunk rotation instead of leading with the arm. Make sure to keep your hips still when you perform this variation.

PREPARATORY STAGE
Kneel on the floor with your shoulders above your wrists, and your hips above your knees. With your gaze down towards the floor, raise your right hand and place it on the side of your head.

STAGE ONE
Inhale as you rotate the body from your waist and trunk, opening your chest and shoulders towards your right side. Look up towards your right elbow.

STAGE TWO
Exhale as you return to the preparatory position of four-point kneeling. Bring your right arm down and look down towards the floor once again. Repeat the sequence 3–6 times, then switch sides.

THREAD THE NEEDLE IN ADDUCTOR STRETCH

This variation has the advantage of stretching the inner thigh muscles, while allowing a good thoracic and upper body stretch. It is a satisfying stretch for the whole body. Don't overdo the stretch if you suffer from pelvic pain.

PREPARATORY STAGE
Start in four-point kneeling, extending your left leg out to the side. Breathe out to thread your left arm underneath your right arm, which will bring your chest and left shoulder towards the floor.

STAGE ONE
Breathe in and open the left arm out and up towards the ceiling. Allow your your trunk to rotate, following with your chest and head. Look up towards your left hand.

STAGE TWO
Bring your left arm back down and thread it again under your right arm. Repeat the sequence then reset to the preparatory four-point kneeling pose.

MERMAID

This stretch lengthens and opens the side of your body while mobilizing the thoracic spine. In performing the Mermaid, you will create space in the ribcage to promote lateral breathing.

KEY

● Primary target muscle

● Secondary target muscle

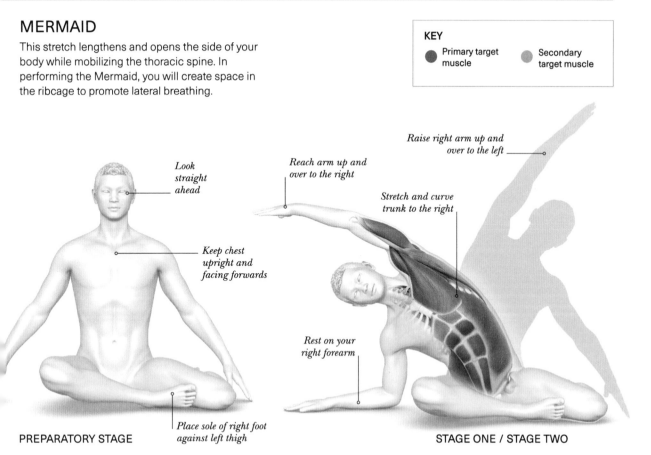

Look straight ahead

Keep chest upright and facing forwards

Place sole of right foot against left thigh

PREPARATORY STAGE

Reach arm up and over to the right

Rest on your right forearm

Raise right arm up and over to the left

Stretch and curve trunk to the right

STAGE ONE / STAGE TWO

PREPARATORY STAGE
Sit upright with your head, neck, spine, and pelvis in neutral and your legs bent to the left side, flexed at the knees. Connect the sole of the right foot with the left thigh. Stretch both arms out by your sides and rest your fingertips lightly on the floor.

STAGE ONE
Breathe in to raise your left arm to the side and over your head. Breathe in to reach the arm up and over to your right side, curving your spine to the right. Slide your right arm along the mat until you rest on your forearm with your palm facing downwards.

STAGE TWO
Return back to the preparatory sitting position, arms once more by your sides. Now raise your right arm up and over to your left, allowing your spine to follow into a left-angled curve.

66 99

Placing the hips in different positions when reaching and rotating can help with multiplanar movement involving the thoracic spine.

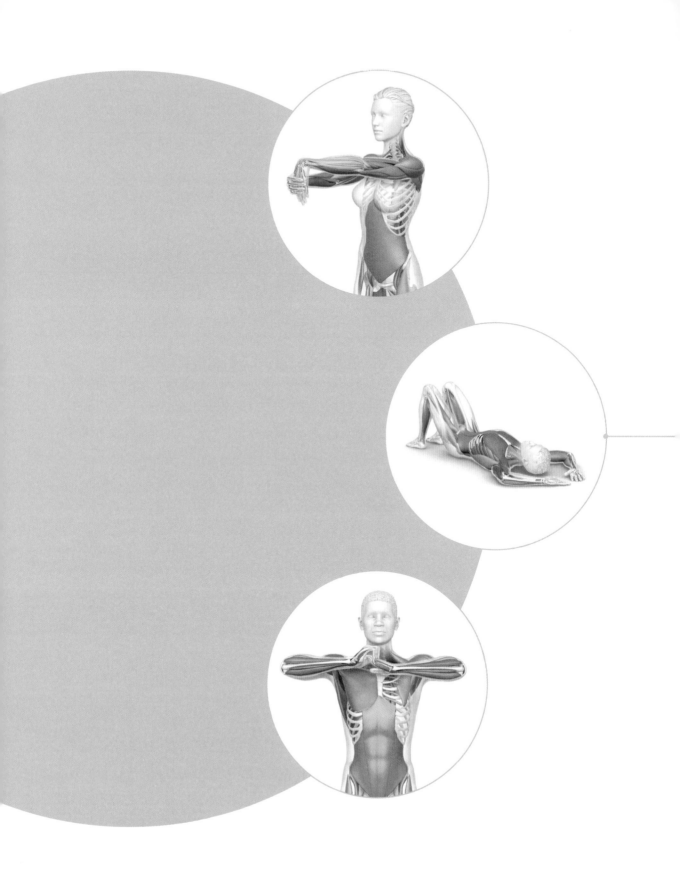

SHOULDER, ARM, AND HAND EXERCISES

The shoulder ranks as the most mobile joint in the body, and upper extremity function is key to successfully completing daily tasks. Range of motion requirements for sports, and activities of daily living, like reaching overhead, require flexibility and strength in both the shoulders and the arms. Wrists and hands are often neglected when it comes to stretching, but it is important to keep them flexible and working correctly. The following exercises help improve mobility in these areas.

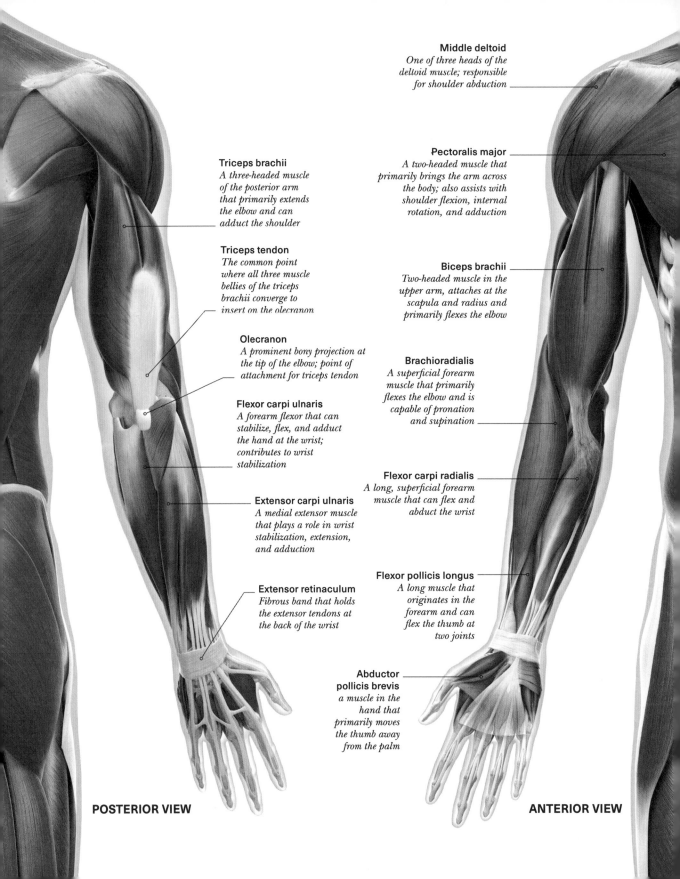

Middle deltoid
One of three heads of the deltoid muscle; responsible for shoulder abduction

Triceps brachii
A three-headed muscle of the posterior arm that primarily extends the elbow and can adduct the shoulder

Triceps tendon
The common point where all three muscle bellies of the triceps brachii converge to insert on the olecranon

Olecranon
A prominent bony projection at the tip of the elbow; point of attachment for triceps tendon

Flexor carpi ulnaris
A forearm flexor that can stabilize, flex, and adduct the hand at the wrist; contributes to wrist stabilization

Extensor carpi ulnaris
A medial extensor muscle that plays a role in wrist stabilization, extension, and adduction

Extensor retinaculum
Fibrous band that holds the extensor tendons at the back of the wrist

Pectoralis major
A two-headed muscle that primarily brings the arm across the body; also assists with shoulder flexion, internal rotation, and adduction

Biceps brachii
Two-headed muscle in the upper arm, attaches at the scapula and radius and primarily flexes the elbow

Brachioradialis
A superficial forearm muscle that primarily flexes the elbow and is capable of pronation and supination

Flexor carpi radialis
A long, superficial forearm muscle that can flex and abduct the wrist

Flexor pollicis longus
A long muscle that originates in the forearm and can flex the thumb at two joints

Abductor pollicis brevis
a muscle in the hand that primarily moves the thumb away from the palm

POSTERIOR VIEW

ANTERIOR VIEW

SHOULDER, ARM, AND HAND OVERVIEW

The muscles of the shoulder, arm, and hand include the serratus anterior, deltoid, rotator cuff muscles, biceps, triceps, forearm flexors and extensors, and intrinsic hand muscles. These important muscles work together to control shoulder and elbow movement, and enable many everyday actions.

The muscles of the shoulder, arm, and hand enable reaching, lifting, gripping, and fine motor skills. The deltoid and rotator cuff muscles help stabilize and move the shoulder joint, allowing for reaching and lifting. The biceps and triceps contribute to elbow motion, which is important for actions such as lifting, pushing, or pulling objects. Forearm flexors and extensors control wrist movements and grip strength. Intrinsic hand muscles enable fine motor skills like writing and manipulation of objects.

Flexibility and strength training can improve joint mobility in the arms, improving function in daily tasks but also in many sports that involve using the arms, such as basketball, tennis, climbing, gymnastics, or swimming.

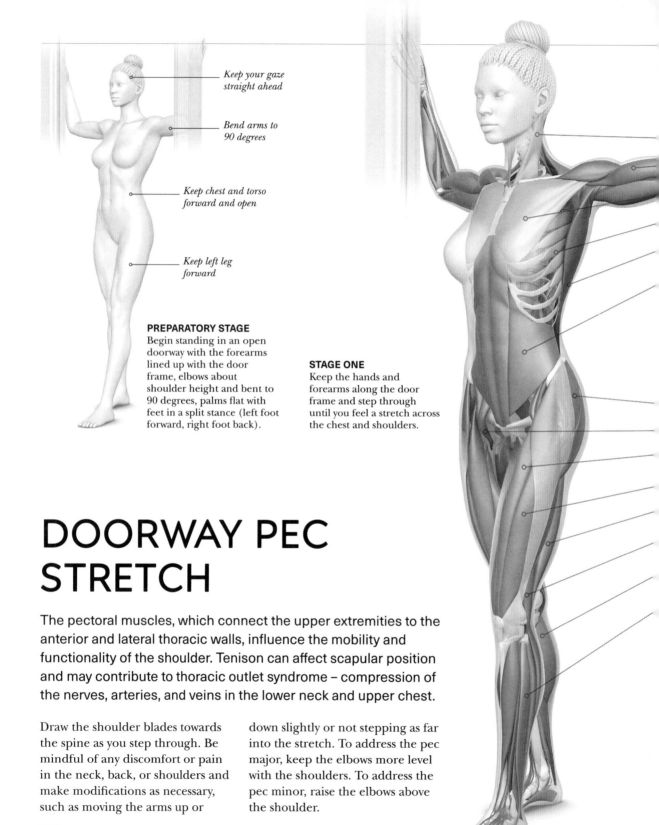

Keep your gaze straight ahead

Bend arms to 90 degrees

Keep chest and torso forward and open

Keep left leg forward

PREPARATORY STAGE
Begin standing in an open doorway with the forearms lined up with the door frame, elbows about shoulder height and bent to 90 degrees, palms flat with feet in a split stance (left foot forward, right foot back).

STAGE ONE
Keep the hands and forearms along the door frame and step through until you feel a stretch across the chest and shoulders.

DOORWAY PEC STRETCH

The pectoral muscles, which connect the upper extremities to the anterior and lateral thoracic walls, influence the mobility and functionality of the shoulder. Tenison can affect scapular position and may contribute to thoracic outlet syndrome – compression of the nerves, arteries, and veins in the lower neck and upper chest.

Draw the shoulder blades towards the spine as you step through. Be mindful of any discomfort or pain in the neck, back, or shoulders and make modifications as necessary, such as moving the arms up or down slightly or not stepping as far into the stretch. To address the pec major, keep the elbows more level with the shoulders. To address the pec minor, raise the elbows above the shoulder.

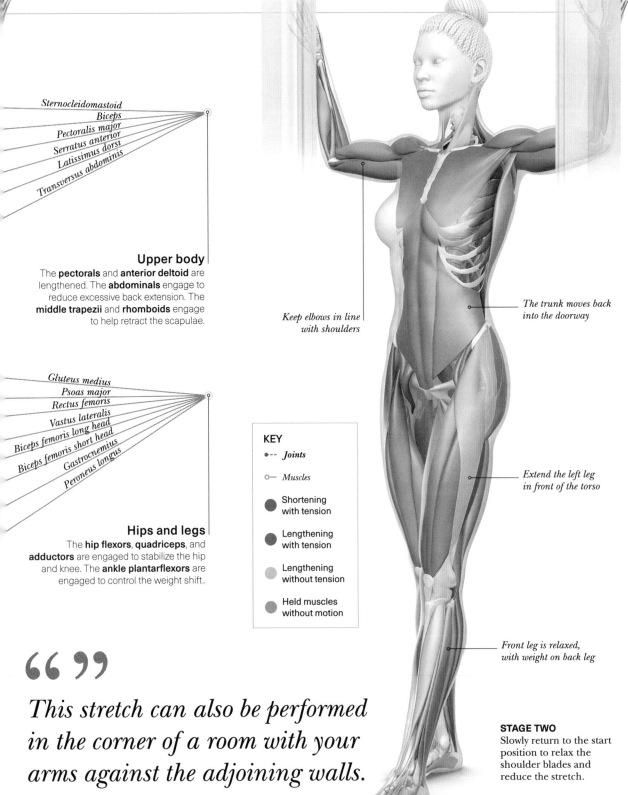

Sternocleidomastoid
Biceps
Pectoralis major
Serratus anterior
Latissimus dorsi
Transversus abdominis

Upper body
The **pectorals** and **anterior deltoid** are lengthened. The **abdominals** engage to reduce excessive back extension. The **middle trapezii** and **rhomboids** engage to help retract the scapulae.

Gluteus medius
Psoas major
Rectus femoris
Vastus lateralis
Biceps femoris long head
Biceps femoris short head
Gastrocnemius
Peroneus longus

Hips and legs
The **hip flexors**, **quadriceps**, and **adductors** are engaged to stabilize the hip and knee. The **ankle plantarflexors** are engaged to control the weight shift..

KEY

•-- *Joints*

○— *Muscles*

● Shortening with tension

● Lengthening with tension

● Lengthening without tension

● Held muscles without motion

Keep elbows in line with shoulders

The trunk moves back into the doorway

Extend the left leg in front of the torso

Front leg is relaxed, with weight on back leg

STAGE TWO
Slowly return to the start position to relax the shoulder blades and reduce the stretch.

66 99

This stretch can also be performed in the corner of a room with your arms against the adjoining walls.

» VARIATIONS

The shoulder is one of the most mobile joints in the body. Opting for various stretches to challenge new positions can help maintain mobility in this area.

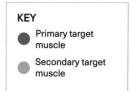

Place right palm and forearm on doorway

Look straight ahead

Chest is open and facing forward

Body faces forwards

PREPARATORY STAGE

Place left leg in front of right in staggered stance

Maintain tall posture with a neutral neck

Shift body forward

STAGE ONE

Bend left knee slightly

PEC MINOR STRETCH

This stretch requires the arm to be slightly higher than the shoulder, due to the angle of the muscle. Try the stretch in a general postural programme, or for shoulder mobility and neck pain relief.

PREPARATORY STAGE
Begin standing next to a doorway with the right forearm and hand rested on it just above shoulder height. Relax your left arm by your side.

STAGE ONE
Gently lean forward, bending your left knee slightly while keeping a tall posture and drawing the shoulder blade towards the spine for a stretch in the chest.

STAGE TWO
Shift your weight back to come out of the stretch. Repeat on the other side.

! Caution

If you feel numbness or tingling in the arm, or neck pain, try lowering the elbow on the doorway. If symptoms persist, consult a professional.

CROSS BODY ARM STRETCH

This is a great shoulder stretch that focusses on the muscles of the posterior shoulder. It can be helpful in addressing shoulder mobility. Perform as part of a daily stretch routine or to address mobility in the shoulders.

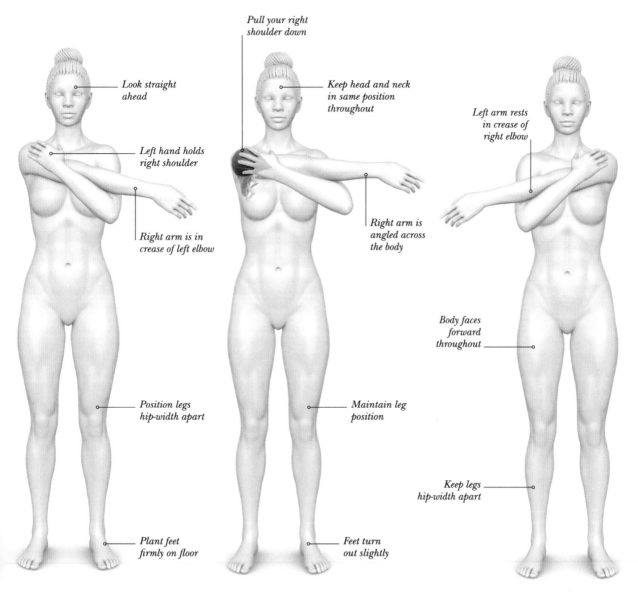

Pull your right shoulder down

Look straight ahead

Left hand holds right shoulder

Right arm is in crease of left elbow

Position legs hip-width apart

Plant feet firmly on floor

Keep head and neck in same position throughout

Right arm is angled across the body

Maintain leg position

Feet turn out slightly

Left arm rests in crease of right elbow

Body faces forward throughout

Keep legs hip-width apart

PREPARATORY STAGE
In a standing position, draw the right arm across your body and hold it in the crease of your left elbow.

STAGE ONE
Holding your right shoulder with your left palm, gently pull the shoulder down so your right arm stretches across the body. Keep your hips square and your body facing forward during the stretch.

STAGE TWO
Relax and repeat on the opposite arm, starting in the preparatory position with the left arm angled down, then pulling on left shoulder so the arm stretches across body.

FLOOR ANGEL

The Floor Angel pec stretch is a simple exercise which targets tension in the pectorals. It also helps open up the shoulders, while engaging the postural muscles that control the scapulae.

The external feedback from the floor on the shoulder blades and hands helps with the quality of scapular retraction and shoulder external rotation. However, this is an adaptable stretch that can also be performed standing against a wall. Use it as part of a daily stretch routine or to improve mobility in the shoulders and reduce any tension in the neck.

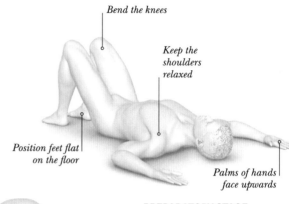

Bend the knees

Keep the shoulders relaxed

Position feet flat on the floor

Palms of hands face upwards

PREPARATORY STAGE
Begin lying on the floor with knees bent and feet flat. Rest your arms on the floor above your head with elbows bent to nearly 90 degrees at shoulder height.

KEY

●-- *Joints*

○— *Muscles*

● Shortening with tension

● Lengthening with tension

● Lengthening without tension

● Held muscles without motion

STAGE ONE
Slide the hands and forearms along the floor and bring the elbows down towards the ribs by pinching the shoulder blades down and back. Your elbows should form a "V" shape.

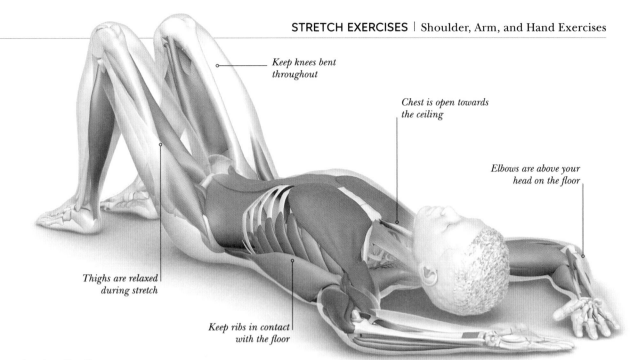

Keep knees bent
throughout

Chest is open towards
the ceiling

Elbows are above your
head on the floor

Thighs are relaxed
during stretch

Keep ribs in contact
with the floor

66 99

The Floor Angel aids postural awareness by targeting muscles of the shoulder blade and rotator cuff.

STAGE TWO

Slide the hands and forearms back upwards towards the head so that the elbows are above the head and the hands are behind it, fingertips facing each other. Return to the preparatory position to repeat the stretch.

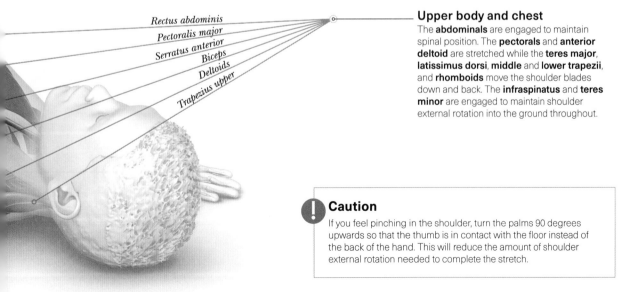

Rectus abdominis
Pectoralis major
Serratus anterior
Biceps
Deltoids
Trapezius upper

Upper body and chest

The **abdominals** are engaged to maintain spinal position. The **pectorals** and **anterior deltoid** are stretched while the **teres major**, **latissimus dorsi**, **middle** and **lower trapezii**, and **rhomboids** move the shoulder blades down and back. The **infraspinatus** and **teres minor** are engaged to maintain shoulder external rotation into the ground throughout.

! Caution

If you feel pinching in the shoulder, turn the palms 90 degrees upwards so that the thumb is in contact with the floor instead of the back of the hand. This will reduce the amount of shoulder external rotation needed to complete the stretch.

WRIST EXTENSION

The simple Wrist Extension exercise helps target tension in the wrists, forearms, and finger flexors. As you don't need any equipment, you can practise it standing or sitting, anywhere, any time.

The muscles of the anterior forearm (flexors) control the wrist and fingers and attach to the medial elbow. Incorporate the Wrist Extension stretch into your daily stretch routine to improve wrist mobility. It may be particularly helpful for those who use their hands often – for example typing, or working in manual labour.

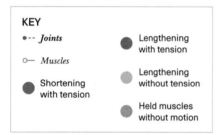

KEY

•-- *Joints*

o— *Muscles*

● Shortening with tension

● Lengthening with tension

● Lengthening without tension

● Held muscles without motion

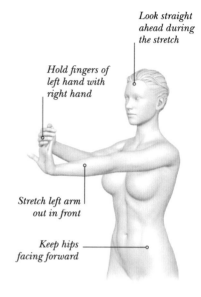

Look straight ahead during the stretch

Hold fingers of left hand with right hand

Stretch left arm out in front

Keep hips facing forward

PREPARATORY STAGE
Begin standing with the left arm stretched out in front, left palm facing upwards, and the right hand holding the fingers of the left hand.

WRIST FLEXION

The Wrist Flexion stretch is easy to perform anywhere and doesn't require any equipment. It helps target tension in the wrist, forearm, and finger extensors.

The muscles of the posterior forearm extensors control the wrist and fingers and attach to the lateral elbow. Incorporate the Wrist Flexion stretch into your daily stretch or to address mobility; you can perform the stretch in tandem with the Wrist Extension stretch.

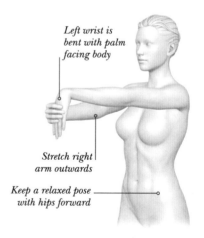

Left wrist is bent with palm facing body

Stretch right arm outwards

Keep a relaxed pose with hips forward

PREPARATORY STAGE
Begin standing with the left arm stretched out in front and the right hand holding the fingers of the left hand, palm towards you, and facing down towards the floor.

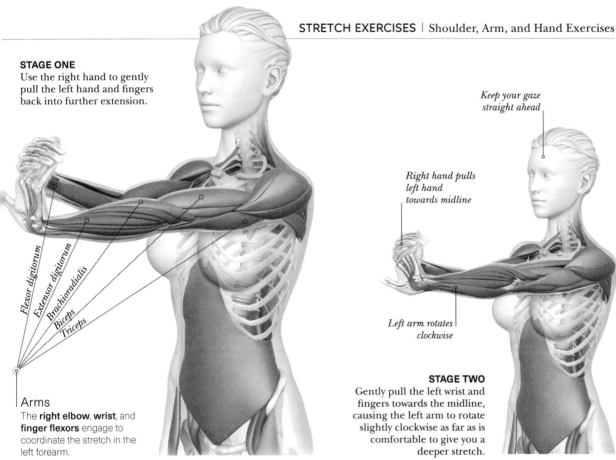

STAGE ONE
Use the right hand to gently pull the left hand and fingers back into further extension.

Flexor digitorum
Extensor digitorum
Brachioradialis
Biceps
Triceps

Arms
The **right elbow**, **wrist**, and **finger flexors** engage to coordinate the stretch in the left forearm.

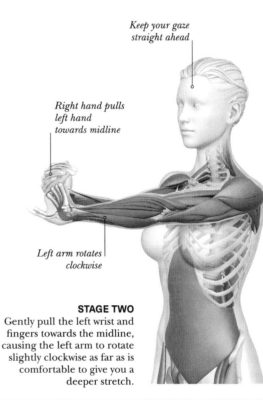

Keep your gaze straight ahead

Right hand pulls left hand towards midline

Left arm rotates clockwise

STAGE TWO
Gently pull the left wrist and fingers towards the midline, causing the left arm to rotate slightly clockwise as far as is comfortable to give you a deeper stretch.

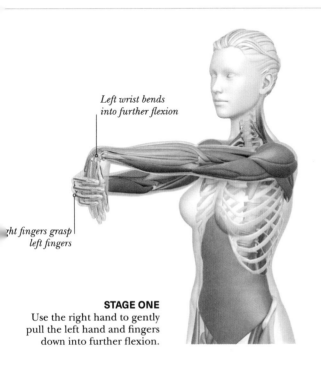

Left wrist bends into further flexion

right fingers grasp left fingers

STAGE ONE
Use the right hand to gently pull the left hand and fingers down into further flexion.

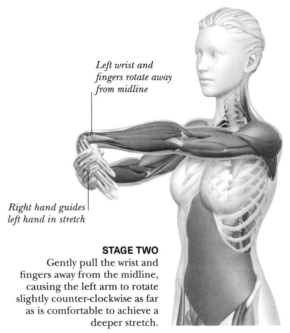

Left wrist and fingers rotate away from midline

Right hand guides left hand in stretch

STAGE TWO
Gently pull the wrist and fingers away from the midline, causing the left arm to rotate slightly counter-clockwise as far as is comfortable to achieve a deeper stretch.

» VARIATIONS

Many activities and sports, such as gymnastics or yoga, require the body to bear weight through the hands and wrists. Practising these variations to provide the necessary mobility in these areas can help reduce injury risk.

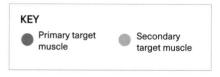
FLOOR WRIST EXTENSION

This is a perfect stretch for those who feel more comfortable exercising on the floor. It targets the muscles of the forearm, with the assistance of the floor, and allows you to choose the pressure imposed.

PREPARATORY STAGE
Begin in four-point kneeling with your palms on the floor, and your fingers pointed towards your knees.

STAGE ONE
Gently sit back towards the heels to feel a comfortable pressure through the fingers and palms, allowing the stretch to occur in the anterior forearm. Make sure the fronts of the elbows are facing forward. Your palms may peel slightly off the floor as you descend.

STAGE TWO
Shift your weight forward again to come out of the stretch.

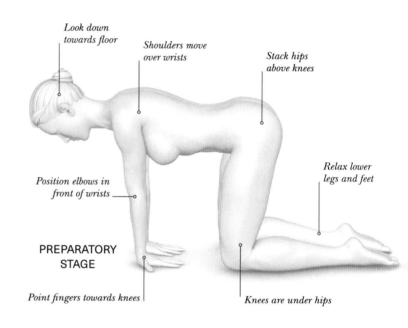

Look down towards floor

Shoulders move over wrists

Stack hips above knees

Position elbows in front of wrists

Relax lower legs and feet

PREPARATORY STAGE

Point fingers towards knees

Knees are under hips

FLOOR WRIST FLEXION

This stretch can be paired with the extension variation to encourage a gentle stretch in the wrist extensors. It targets the muscles of the forearm, with the freedom to apply as much pressure as you can tolerate.

PREPARATORY STAGE
Begin on your hands and knees with the wrists flexed, backs of the hands on the floor, and shoulders in front of hands.

STAGE ONE
Gently shift your weight back slightly to feel a stretch into greater flexion. Keep the elbows rotated to face forwards.

STAGE TWO
Shift the body forward again to come out of the stretch.

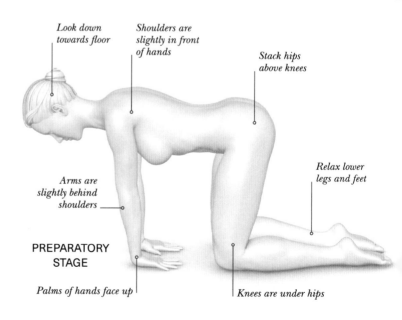

Look down towards floor

Shoulders are slightly in front of hands

Stack hips above knees

Arms are slightly behind shoulders

Relax lower legs and feet

PREPARATORY STAGE

Palms of hands face up

Knees are under hips

" "

The intensity of the stretch can be modified by the range of motion and amount of weight you place through the wrists.

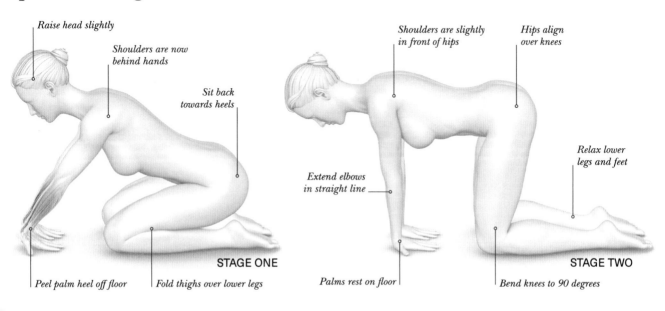

Raise head slightly

Shoulders are now behind hands

Sit back towards heels

STAGE ONE

Peel palm heel off floor

Fold thighs over lower legs

Shoulders are slightly in front of hips

Hips align over knees

Relax lower legs and feet

Extend elbows in straight line

STAGE TWO

Palms rest on floor

Bend knees to 90 degrees

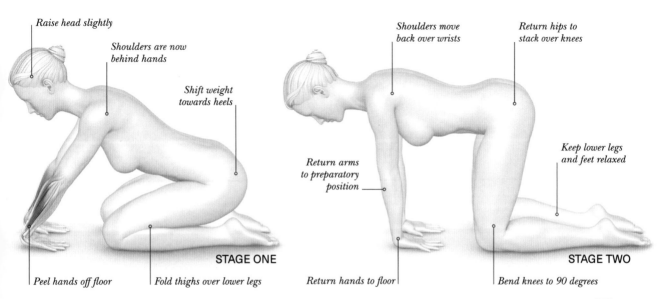

Raise head slightly

Shoulders are now behind hands

Shift weight towards heels

STAGE ONE

Peel hands off floor

Fold thighs over lower legs

Shoulders move back over wrists

Return hips to stack over knees

Keep lower legs and feet relaxed

Return arms to preparatory position

STAGE TWO

Return hands to floor

Bend knees to 90 degrees

111

LUMBRICAL STRETCH

This hand stretch targets tension in the hand and between the metacarpophalangeal (MCP) joints, commonly known as the large knuckles. The lumbricals originate from the tendons of the deep finger flexor in the palm. In linking flexor tendons with extensor tendons, they can flex the MCP joints while extending the finger.

Because the lumbricals contribute to grip strength, the Lumbrical Stretch may be especially helpful for those who use their hands to perform fine motor tasks, such as typists, artists, or musicians. It can also be helpful for those who use their hands a lot – for example in manual work or rock climbing. Use it to address fatigue or tension in the hand or as part of a greater mobility programme.

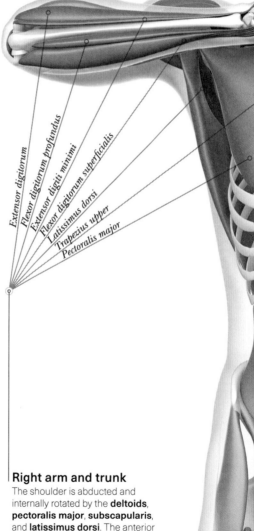

Extensor digitorum
Flexor digitorum profundus
Extensor digiti minimi
Flexor digitorum superficialis
Latissimus dorsi
Trapezius upper
Pectoralis major

Right arm and trunk
The shoulder is abducted and internally rotated by the **deltoids**, **pectoralis major**, **subscapularis**, and **latissimus dorsi**. The anterior forearm and hand muscles engage. The **abdominals** and **spinal extensors** stabilize the trunk.

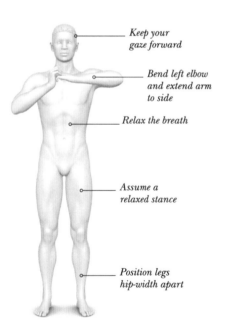

Keep your gaze forward

Bend left elbow and extend arm to side

Relax the breath

Assume a relaxed stance

Position legs hip-width apart

PREPARATORY STAGE
Begin standing with the right hand cupped over the left fingers and knuckles.

KEY

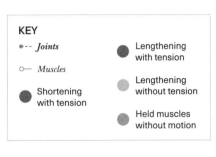

•--- *Joints*

○— *Muscles*

● Shortening with tension

● Lengthening with tension

● Lengthening without tension

● Held muscles without motion

> " "
> *There are four lumbrical muscles, each associated with one finger from digits two to five.*

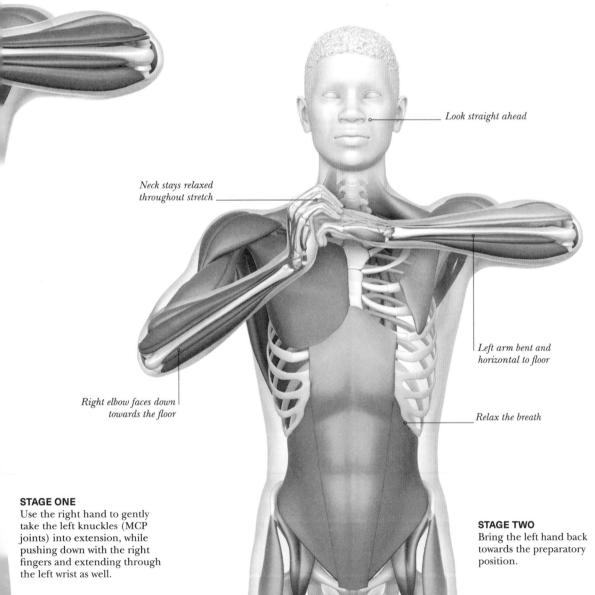

Look straight ahead

Neck stays relaxed throughout stretch

Left arm bent and horizontal to floor

Right elbow faces down towards the floor

Relax the breath

STAGE ONE
Use the right hand to gently take the left knuckles (MCP joints) into extension, while pushing down with the right fingers and extending through the left wrist as well.

STAGE TWO
Bring the left hand back towards the preparatory position.

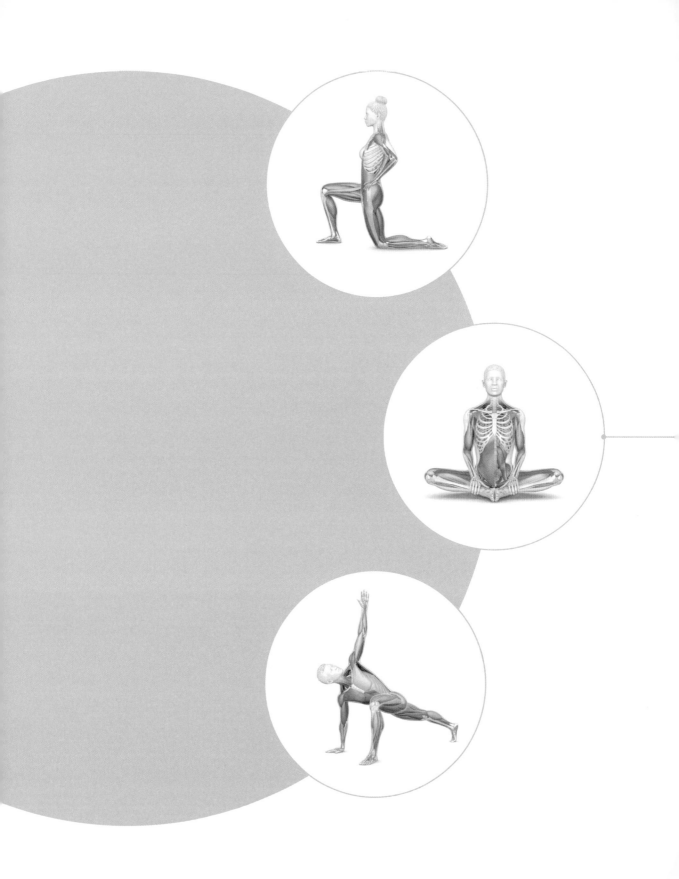

HIP EXERCISES

The ball-and-socket hip joint plays a crucial role in providing stability and support to the upper body and carrying out weightbearing activities, while having the ability to move in all planes of motion. This section highlights exercises that target the hip muscles and aim to improve range of motion in this important joint.

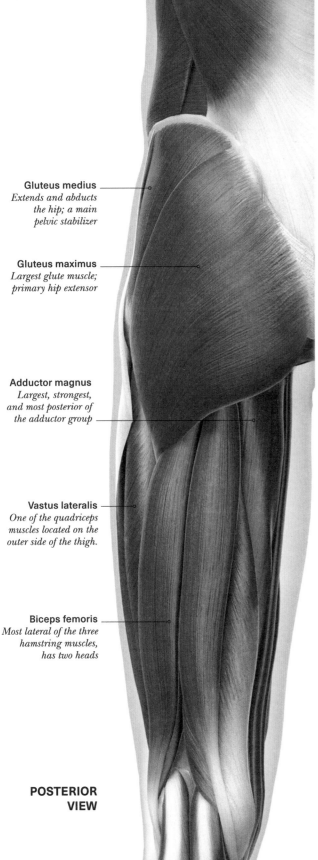

Gluteus medius
Extends and abducts the hip; a main pelvic stabilizer

Gluteus maximus
Largest glute muscle; primary hip extensor

Adductor magnus
Largest, strongest, and most posterior of the adductor group

Vastus lateralis
One of the quadriceps muscles located on the outer side of the thigh.

Biceps femoris
Most lateral of the three hamstring muscles, has two heads

POSTERIOR VIEW

Internal oblique
Abdominal muscles located on the sides of the torso, deep to the external obliques

Gluteus minimus
Smaller glute muscle, located deep to gluteus medius

Psoas major
Joins with the iliacus to form the iliopsoas, acts as a primary hip flexor can also flex the trunk

Pectineus
Helps connect the ante and medial thigh; can adduct, and internally rotate the hip

Adductor longus
Quadrangular muscle helps connect the anteri and medial thigh; can adduct, and internally rotate the hip

Gracilis
Long, thin, superficia muscle that aids in flexing and adduction at the hip and knee

Sartorius
The longest muscle of the body; crosses the hi and knee joints; can flex and rotate both

Vastus lateralis
The most lateral of the quadriceps muscles; considered to be the strongest of the group

ANTERIOR VIEW

HIP OVERVIEW

The primary muscles of the hip and thigh include the gluteal muscles (gluteus maximus, medius, and minimus), ilacus and psoas major, quadriceps (rectus femoris, vastus lateralis, vastus medialis, and vastus intermedius), hamstrings (biceps femoris, semitendinosus, and semimembranosus), and adductor muscles.

The muscles around the hips have different actions that help with multidirectional movement and provide stability for the pelvis and hips. Muscles like the iliopsoas and rectus femoris help with hip flexion, while others, like the glutes and hamstrings, help with hip extension.

The hip abductors, such as the gluteus medius and tensor fasciae latae, keep the pelvis stable when standing on one leg. The adductors contribute to many movements beyond adduction, while several muscles contribute to hip rotation. The quadriceps extend the knee, and the hamstrings help flex it and assist in hip extension, which is important for activities like running, football, and weightlifting.

QUADRUPED ROCKBACK

This stretch is a great way to facilitate hip mobility in a pose that is easy for beginners to adopt. Hip flexion mobility is achieved by rocking the pelvis and trunk backwards while keeping the hands and knees fixed on the floor.

This is a gentle, low weight-bearing stretch suitable for beginners or those who are in early-phase hip rehabilitation. It can help to gradually increase range of motion in the hips by moving the pelvis on the hip joint, which may be easier for those with limitations in active movement.

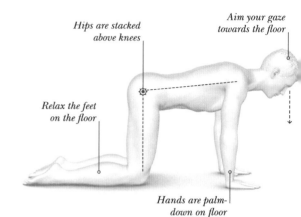

Hips are stacked above knees

Aim your gaze towards the floor

Relax the feet on the floor

Hands are palm-down on floor

PREPARATORY STAGE
Begin in the four-point kneeling position with the shoulders above the wrists, the hips above the knees, and head and neck in line. Keep your spine neutral – the middle, comfortable zone between fully flexed and fully extended.

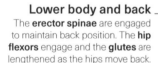

Lower body and back
The **erector spinae** are engaged to maintain back position. The **hip flexors** engage and the **glutes** are lengthened as the hips move back.

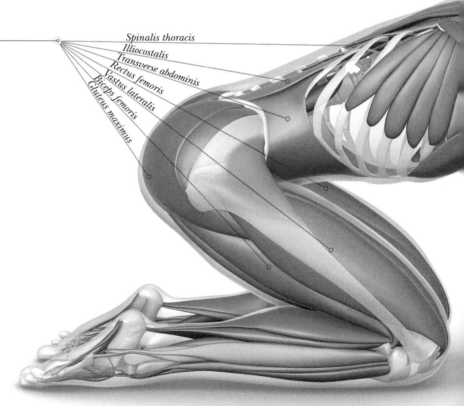

Spinalis thoracis
Illiocostalis
Transverse abdominis
Rectus femoris
Vastus lateralis
Biceps femoris
Gluteus maximus

STAGE ONE
Gently push back into the hips, until you can feel a stretch in and around them. Keep the back in a comfortable position as pelvic positioning may affect the depth of the stretch; stay within a comfortable zone and hold for a few seconds.

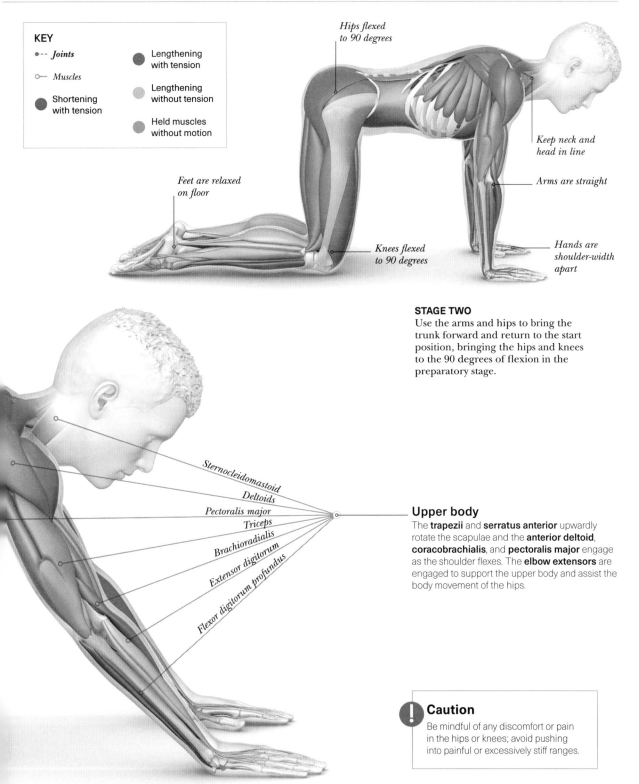

KEY

•-- *Joints*

○— *Muscles*

● Shortening with tension

● Lengthening with tension

● Lengthening without tension

● Held muscles without motion

Hips flexed to 90 degrees

Keep neck and head in line

Arms are straight

Feet are relaxed on floor

Knees flexed to 90 degrees

Hands are shoulder-width apart

STAGE TWO
Use the arms and hips to bring the trunk forward and return to the start position, bringing the hips and knees to the 90 degrees of flexion in the preparatory stage.

Sternocleidomastoid

Deltoids

Pectoralis major

Triceps

Brachioradialis

Extensor digitorum

Flexor digitorum profundus

Upper body
The **trapezii** and **serratus anterior** upwardly rotate the scapulae and the **anterior deltoid**, **coracobrachialis**, and **pectoralis major** engage as the shoulder flexes. The **elbow extensors** are engaged to support the upper body and assist the body movement of the hips.

! Caution
Be mindful of any discomfort or pain in the hips or knees; avoid pushing into painful or excessively stiff ranges.

» VARIATIONS

The Rockback variations present ways to involve other muscle groups while moving into hip flexion. These stretches are great dynamic options to include before performing lower body sport or activity.

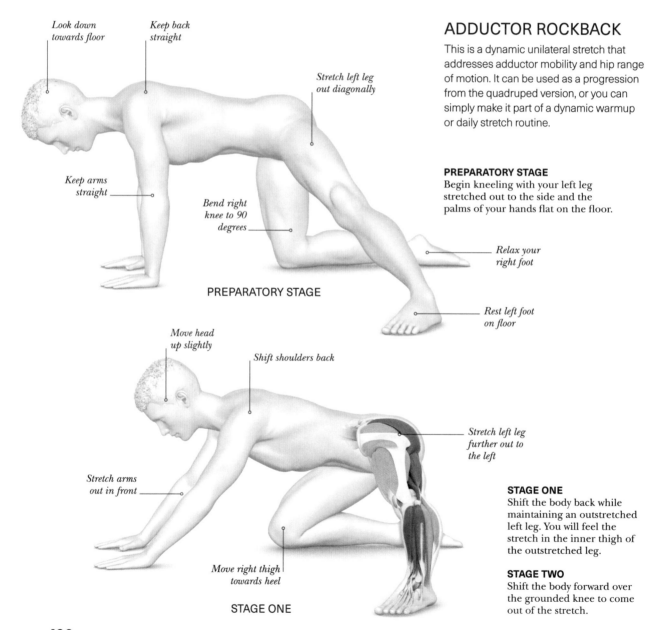

Look down towards floor

Keep back straight

Stretch left leg out diagonally

Keep arms straight

Bend right knee to 90 degrees

Relax your right foot

Rest left foot on floor

PREPARATORY STAGE

Move head up slightly

Shift shoulders back

Stretch left leg further out to the left

Stretch arms out in front

Move right thigh towards heel

STAGE ONE

ADDUCTOR ROCKBACK

This is a dynamic unilateral stretch that addresses adductor mobility and hip range of motion. It can be used as a progression from the quadruped version, or you can simply make it part of a dynamic warmup or daily stretch routine.

PREPARATORY STAGE
Begin kneeling with your left leg stretched out to the side and the palms of your hands flat on the floor.

STAGE ONE
Shift the body back while maintaining an outstretched left leg. You will feel the stretch in the inner thigh of the outstretched leg.

STAGE TWO
Shift the body forward over the grounded knee to come out of the stretch.

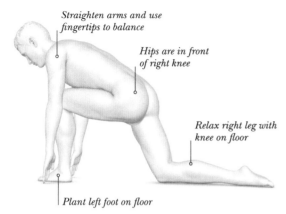

Straighten arms and use fingertips to balance

Hips are in front of right knee

Relax right leg with knee on floor

Plant left foot on floor

PREPARATORY STAGE

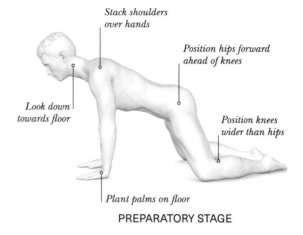

Stack shoulders over hands

Position hips forward ahead of knees

Look down towards floor

Position knees wider than hips

Plant palms on floor

PREPARATORY STAGE

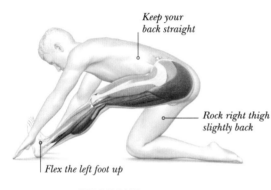

Keep your back straight

Rock right thigh slightly back

Flex the left foot up

STAGE ONE

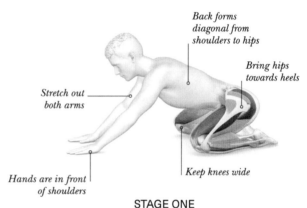

Back forms diagonal from shoulders to hips

Bring hips towards heels

Stretch out both arms

Hands are in front of shoulders

Keep knees wide

STAGE ONE

HAMSTRING ROCKBACK

This dynamic hamstring stretch allows hip flexion and knee extension to occur in the target leg – in this case, the left leg. It is a great stretch for those who practise sports such as running that put a lot of demand on the legs.

PREPARATORY STAGE
Begin in a half-kneel position with your left foot and right knee on the floor. Place your fingertips or hands on the floor for support and flex your trunk forward.

STAGE ONE
Shift your body back while extending the left knee, keeping the back straight and hands on the floor. Flex the left foot up to balance on the left heel, to feel a good stretch in the left hamstring.

STAGE TWO
Shift the body forward to come out of the stretch.

FROG ROCKBACK

This is a dynamic stretch that targets hip abduction and external rotation while stretching the inner thigh muscles. It is a bilateral exercise that can be done as part of a hip mobility routine or warmup.

PREPARATORY STAGE
Begin on your hands and knees with palms flat and knees wider than the hips. Allow your toes to touch behind you.

STAGE ONE
Shift back into a deep stretch, bringing your hips towards your heels and maintaining the wide knee position.

STAGE TWO
Shift the body forward to come out of the stretch.

HALF-KNEEL HIP FLEXOR ROCK

This exercise works to dynamically stretch the anterior hip, including the quadriceps and illiopsoas. The half-kneel position makes the lunging movement easier.

Bending the knee of the rear leg lengthens the quad muscle across the knee joint, and moving the hip into extension increases the stretch across its proximal attachment. This dynamic stretch is also different from its static counterpart in that rocking achieves motion in the front hip and ankle, as well as achieving a stretch in the rear leg. It can be used as a lower body warmup.

> **! Caution**
> Tuck the tailbone slightly and remain in control of the stretch to reduce excessive lumbar extension. If you experience any hip or back pain with the motion, modify the range of motion or opt for a static stretch.

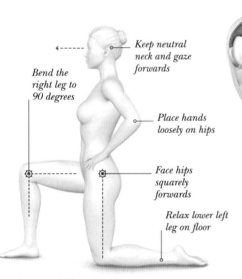

Keep neutral neck and gaze forwards

Bend the right leg to 90 degrees

Place hands loosely on hips

Face hips squarely forwards

Relax lower left leg on floor

PREPARATORY STAGE
Begin in the half-kneeling position with your left knee bent on the floor and your right knee bent in front, right foot flat on the floor. Keep your spine neutral and your gaze forward.

122

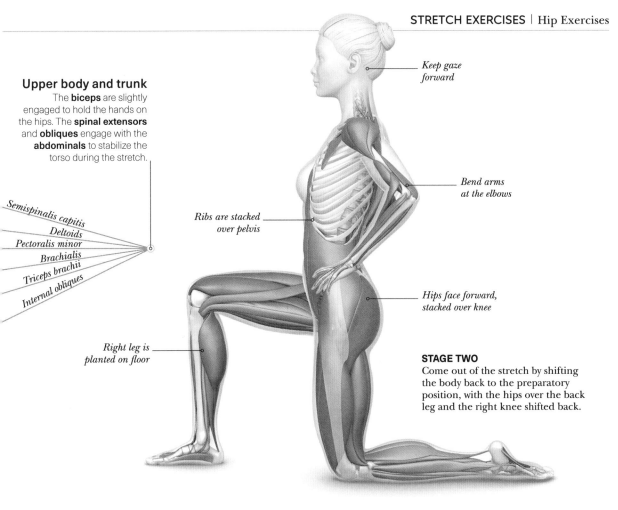

Keep gaze forward

Upper body and trunk

The **biceps** are slightly engaged to hold the hands on the hips. The **spinal extensors** and **obliques** engage with the **abdominals** to stabilize the torso during the stretch.

Semispinalis capitis
Deltoids
Pectoralis minor
Brachialis
Triceps brachii
Internal obliques

Bend arms at the elbows

Ribs are stacked over pelvis

Hips face forward, stacked over knee

Right leg is planted on floor

STAGE TWO

Come out of the stretch by shifting the body back to the preparatory position, with the hips over the back leg and the right knee shifted back.

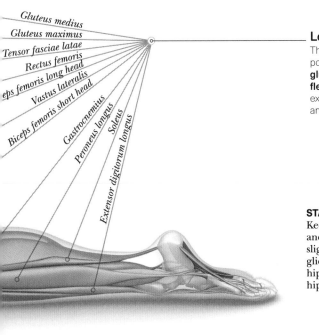

Gluteus medius
Gluteus maximus
Tensor fasciae latae
Rectus femoris
eps femoris long head
Vastus lateralis
Biceps femoris short head
Gastrocnemius
Peroneus longus
Soleus
Extensor digitorum longus

Lower body

The **abdominals** contract to posteriorly tilt the pelvis, and the **glutes** engage. The **left hip flexors** are stretched as the hip is extended, while the **hamstrings** and **gastrocnemius** are relaxed.

STAGE ONE

Keeping the hands on the hips and the hips squared forwards, slightly tilt your tailbone and glide forward to stretch the back hip into extension and the front hip into flexion.

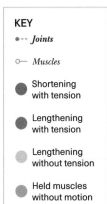

KEY
- •-- *Joints*
- ○— *Muscles*
- Shortening with tension
- Lengthening with tension
- Lengthening without tension
- Held muscles without motion

123

» VARIATIONS

The hip muscle is influenced by many muscle groups, including the hip extensors, flexors, abductors, and adductors. The Hip Flexor Rock series of variations can be done in a sequence to address mobility in both hips.

Caution
Make modifications if you experience any discomfort or pain in the hip, back, or knees. These variations should feel like comfortable movements through both hips.

DIAGONAL FLEXOR ROCK

This variation allows a greater dynamic stretch from the inner thigh and groin muscles, as the hip is positioned about 45 degrees away from the midline prior to the forward rock.

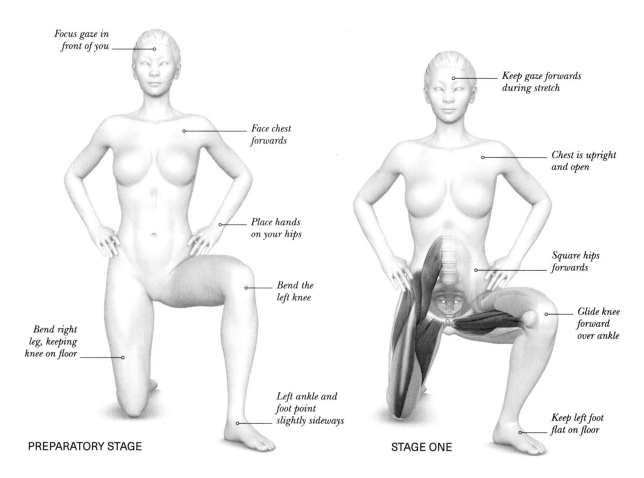

Focus gaze in front of you

Face chest forwards

Place hands on your hips

Bend the left knee

Bend right leg, keeping knee on floor

Left ankle and foot point slightly sideways

PREPARATORY STAGE

Keep gaze forwards during stretch

Chest is upright and open

Square hips forwards

Glide knee forward over ankle

Keep left foot flat on floor

STAGE ONE

PREPARATORY STAGE
Begin in the half-kneeling position with the knees bent to 90 degrees and the left leg slightly to the left of the midline. Place your hands on your hips and keep your spine neutral and gaze forward.

STAGE ONE
Keeping the hands on the hips and the hips squared forwards, slightly tuck in the tailbone and glide forward over the left ankle to stretch the back hip into extension and the front hip into flexion.

STAGE TWO
Shift your weight back over the kneeling leg to come out of the stretch.

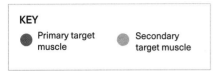

KEY
● Primary target muscle
● Secondary target muscle

The adductor group of muscles assist with these hip movements and undergo a stretch on both sides with each variation.

LATERAL FLEXOR ROCK

This variation provides a dynamic stretch from the inner thigh and groin muscles, as the hip is positioned laterally from the midline prior to the forward rock. It is a great exercise to help open the hips and improve dynamic mobility of the adductor group of muscles.

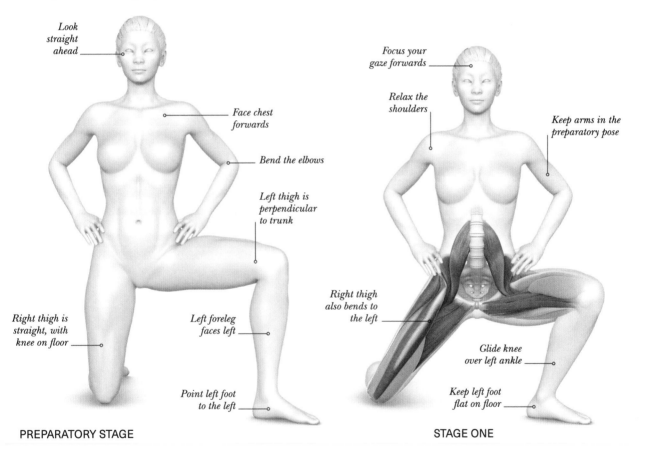

Look straight ahead

Face chest forwards

Bend the elbows

Left thigh is perpendicular to trunk

Right thigh is straight, with knee on floor

Left foreleg faces left

Point left foot to the left

PREPARATORY STAGE

Focus your gaze forwards

Relax the shoulders

Keep arms in the preparatory pose

Right thigh also bends to the left

Glide knee over left ankle

Keep left foot flat on floor

STAGE ONE

PREPARATORY STAGE
Begin in the half-kneeling position with the knees bent at 90 degrees and the right leg pointed away from the midline, completely abducted. Keep your spine neutral and your gaze forward.

STAGE ONE
Keeping your hands on your hips and the hips squared forwards, slightly tuck in your tailbone and glide out over the left ankle. This will stretch the back hip into extension/abduction, and the front hip into flexion/abduction.

STAGE TWO
Shift your weight back over the kneeling leg to come out of the stretch.

GARLAND SQUAT

This squat hold can help to open up the hips, stretch the ankles, and lengthen the pelvic floor. It can be used with or without support and is a good way to help progress range of motion into a deep squat.

If you can't reach the bottom of the Garland Squat comfortably to start with, you can set a target underneath you, like a yoga block, as a stopping point. Using the elbows to help open up the knees provides some outward pressure at each knee, allowing for hip external rotation at the bottom of the range. Practise the squat as part of a daily stretch routine or to address mobility in hips, knees, and ankles in a warmup.

> **⚠ Caution**
> Avoid pushing into any hip pinching or excessive stiffness. Hip joints come in a variety of shapes and sizes and structural variations may limit range of motion. While a new stretch may feel novel, modify for any excessive discomfort.

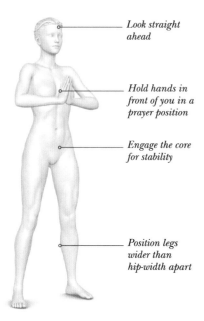

— *Look straight ahead*

— *Hold hands in front of you in a prayer position*

— *Engage the core for stability*

— *Position legs wider than hip-width apart*

PREPARATORY STAGE
Begin standing with feet slightly wider than hips, and pointed outwards slightly.

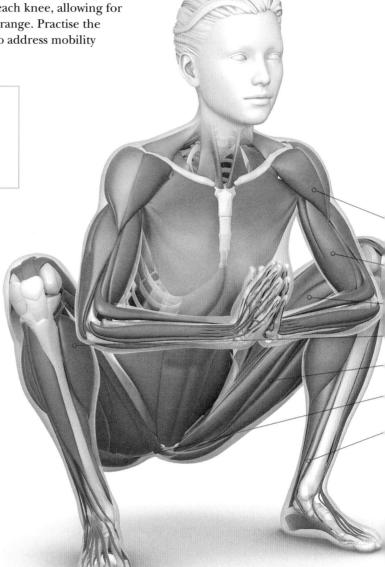

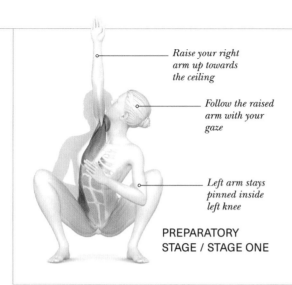

Raise your right arm up towards the ceiling

Follow the raised arm with your gaze

Left arm stays pinned inside left knee

PREPARATORY STAGE / STAGE ONE

VARIATION: ALTERNATING ARM REACH

PREPARATORY STAGE
Begin in the stage 1 of the Garland Squat, at the bottom of your squat, hands prayer position in front of you.

STAGE ONE
Reach the right arm up towards the ceiling, following with the head and neck, while keeping the spine tall and the left arm pinned inside the left knee.

STAGE TWO
Return the right hand down to the inside of the right knee, and repeat the reach with the left arm.

Arms and legs
The **wrist flexors** are lengthened, while the **elbow flexors** and **shoulder abductors** engage. The **glutes** and **adductors** are lengthened with tension. The **ankle plantarflexors** and **dorsiflexors** are also engaged.

Deltoids
Biceps
Sartorius
Gastrocnemius
Semimembranosus
Gluteus maximus
Flexor digitorum longus

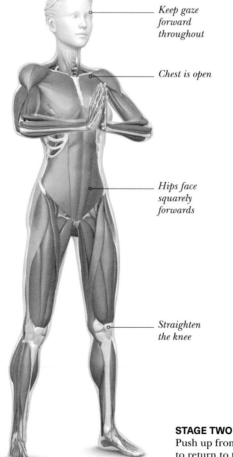

Keep gaze forward throughout

Chest is open

Hips face squarely forwards

Straighten the knee

KEY

●--- *Joints*

○— *Muscles*

● Shortening with tension

● Lengthening with tension

● Lengthening without tension

● Held muscles without motion

STAGE ONE
Lower into a deep squat, placing the elbows on the insides of the knees, so they are adding pressure in an outwards motion as if to prise the hips open. If desired, shift weight from right to left.

STAGE TWO
Push up from the floor to return to the original standing position.

127

FIGURE 4 STRETCH

Performed lying on the floor, this is a great stretch to address external rotation by specifically targeting the glute complex and the hip rotators. It can be helpful to relieve tension in the hip.

Practise the Figure 4 Stretch as a hip mobility exercise or to reduce tension in the glutes that may be contributing to other discomfort, including sciatic pain. The main position on the floor allows for back comfort, whereas the seated variation is a good substitute and can be performed while sitting at a desk. This stretch often is included in programmes that aim to improve hip mobility.

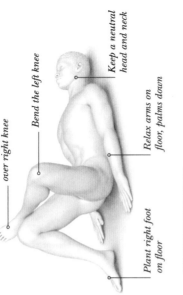

Cross left ankle over right knee

Bend the left knee

Keep a neutral head and neck

Relax arms on floor, palms down

Plant right foot on floor

PREPARATORY STAGE
Begin lying on your back, arms relaxed on the floor, with your left ankle crossed over your right knee.

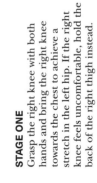

STAGE ONE
Grasp the right knee with both hands and bring the right knee towards the chest to achieve a stretch in the left hip. If the right knee feels uncomfortable, hold the back of the right thigh instead.

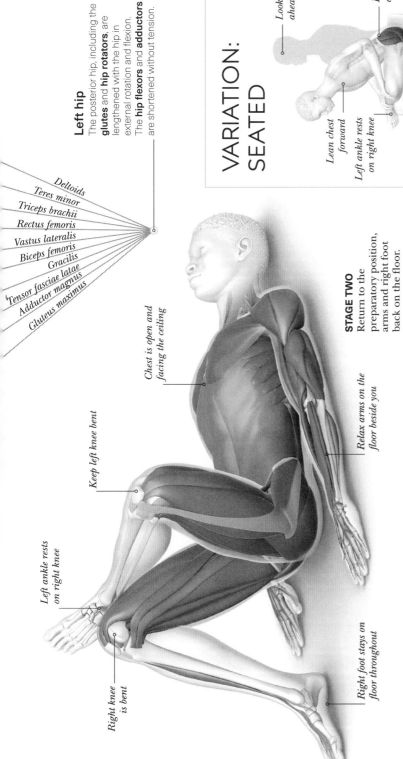

Left hip

The posterior hip, including the **glutes** and **hip rotators**, are lengthened with the hip in external rotation and flexion. The **hip flexors** and **adductors** are shortened without tension.

Deltoids
Teres minor
Triceps brachii
Rectus femoris
Vastus lateralis
Biceps femoris
Gracilis
Tensor fasciae latae
Adductor magnus
Gluteus maximus

Chest is open and facing the ceiling

Keep left knee bent

Left ankle rests on right knee

Right knee is bent

Relax arms on the floor beside you

Right foot stays on floor throughout

STAGE TWO
Return to the preparatory position, arms and right foot back on the floor.

KEY

- ● -- *Joints*
- ○— *Muscles*

Shortening with tension

Lengthening with tension

Lengthening without tension

Held muscles without motion

"

There are six deep hip rotators that underlie the larger, superficial gluteal muscles, and these mainly extend and abduct the hip.

VARIATION: SEATED

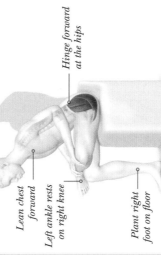

Look straight ahead to start

Hinge forward at the hips

Lean chest forward

Left ankle rests on right knee

Plant right foot on floor

PREPARATORY STAGE
Begin seated with your left ankle crossed over your right knee, hands resting lightly on the knee and ankle of the left leg.

STAGE ONE
With a tall, straight spine, hinge forward at the hips to achieve a stretch in the left hip.

STAGE TWO
Return to the preparatory position.

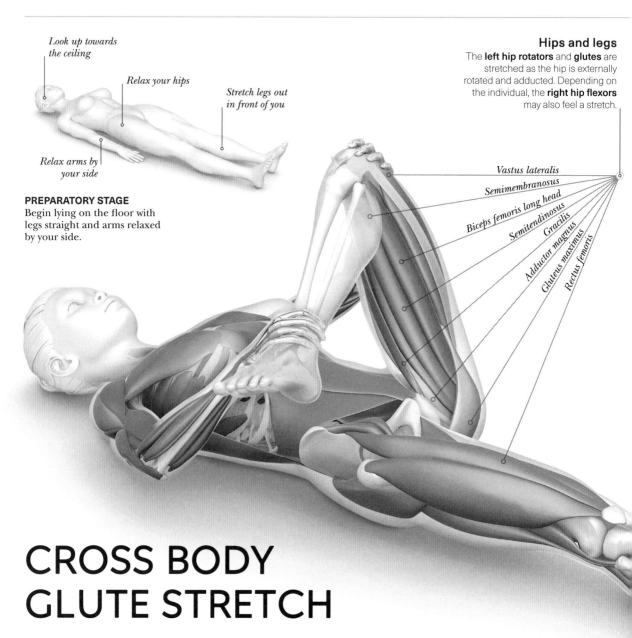

Look up towards
the ceiling

Relax your hips

Stretch legs out
in front of you

Relax arms by
your side

PREPARATORY STAGE
Begin lying on the floor with
legs straight and arms relaxed
by your side.

Hips and legs
The **left hip rotators** and **glutes** are
stretched as the hip is externally
rotated and adducted. Depending on
the individual, the **right hip flexors**
may also feel a stretch.

Vastus lateralis
Semimembranosus
Biceps femoris long head
Semitendinosus
Gracilis
Adductor magnus
Gluteus maximus
Rectus femoris

CROSS BODY GLUTE STRETCH

This stretch is commonly used to target the posterior glute complex and
hip rotators. It can be used as a simple hip mobility exercise or to reduce
tension in the glute that may be causing discomfort in the hip region.

The angle of pull in the Cross Body Glute Stretch is
slightly different from the Figure 4 Stretch (see p.
128). It also calls for a different range of motion in
the hip. The main floor position allows for back
comfort, but if you may prefer to try the the seated
modification if you feel more comfortable sitting on
a chair. You can also practise this variation during a
work day, sitting at a desk. Move into the stretch
gradually and hold at the point where you feel a
good stretch in the glute.

KEY

- ●-- *Joints*
- ○— *Muscles*
- ● Shortening with tension
- ● Lengthening with tension
- ○ Lengthening without tension
- ● Held muscles without motion

! Caution

Remember, structural variations in the hip may limit individual range of motion. Attempt the stretch in tolerable angles.

VARIATION: SEATED

Look straight ahead

Keep your chest upwards

Hold left knee with both hands

Plant right leg on floor

Pull left knee towards right shoulder

PREPARATORY STAGE

Begin seated with your left ankle crossed diagonally over your right knee. Grasp your left knee with both hands.

STAGE ONE

Keeping your spine tall and straight, pull the left knee towards the opposite shoulder to achieve a stretch in the posterior hip. Return to the preparatory position.

Keep your gaze upwards

Pull knee with your left hand

Externally rotate the left hip

Pull on the shin with your right hand

Right leg stays relaxed on floor

Right foot faces upwards

STAGE TWO

Using the arms, pull the hip towards the midline to achieve a stretch in the posterior hip.

STAGE ONE

Bring the left hip up with slight hip external rotation, placing the left hand on the knee and the right hand on the lower shin.

66 99

This glute stretch is suitable for those with limited hip external rotation mobility.

FIGURE 4 HIP INTERNAL ROTATION STRETCH

This is a great stretch for the hips, and it also offers some gentle rotation to the lumbar spine. The mild stretch into hip internal rotation, in a less flexed hip position, can be helpful for people who lack comfortable flexion and internal rotation range of motion.

Hip internal rotation mobility is necessary for daily movement such as getting in and out of vehicles and change of direction in sport. Lacking hip internal rotation may contribute to limitations in hip function.

This simple exercise can help relieve lower back tension while gently stretching the hip. Use control in the stretch, and vary the hip flexion angle by moving the left foot further away or elevating it.

> **! Caution**
> If you experience pain with hip flexion, internal rotation, and adduction, reduce the range of motion in the stretch.

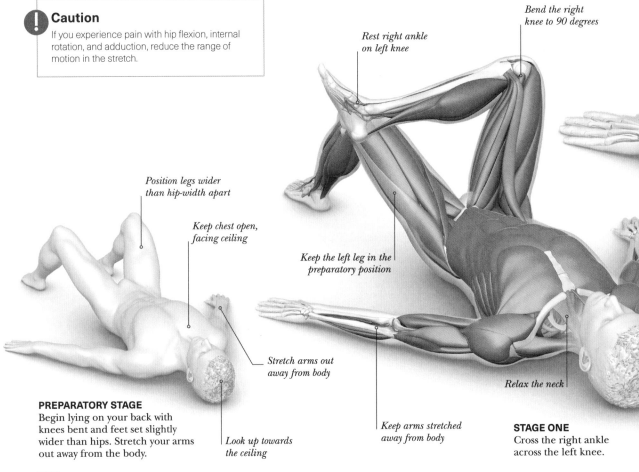

Bend the right knee to 90 degrees

Rest right ankle on left knee

Position legs wider than hip-width apart

Keep chest open, facing ceiling

Keep the left leg in the preparatory position

Stretch arms out away from body

Relax the neck

PREPARATORY STAGE
Begin lying on your back with knees bent and feet set slightly wider than hips. Stretch your arms out away from the body.

Look up towards the ceiling

Keep arms stretched away from body

STAGE ONE
Cross the right ankle across the left knee.

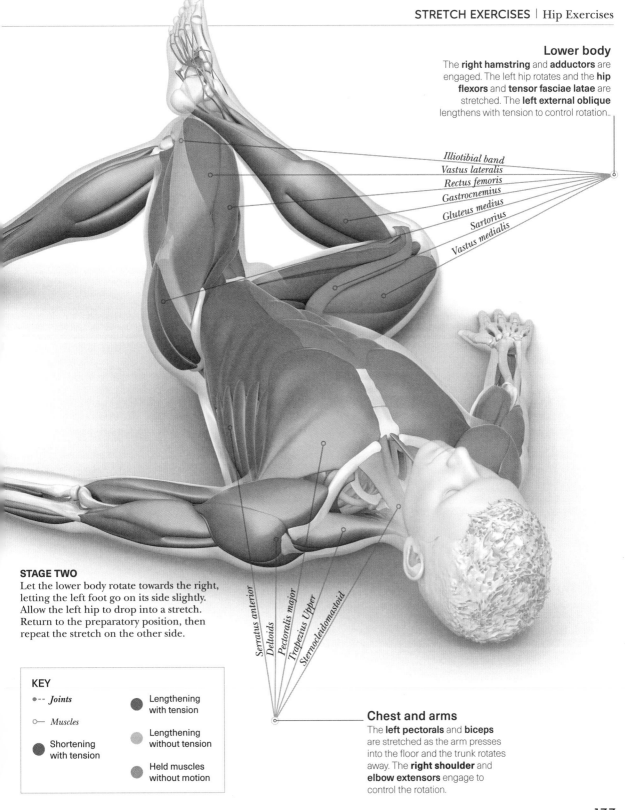

Lower body

The **right hamstring** and **adductors** are engaged. The left hip rotates and the **hip flexors** and **tensor fasciae latae** are stretched. The **left external oblique** lengthens with tension to control rotation..

Illiotibial band
Vastus lateralis
Rectus femoris
Gastrocnemius
Gluteus medius
Sartorius
Vastus medialis

Serratus anterior
Deltoids
Pectoralis major
Trapezius Upper
Sternocleidomastoid

STAGE TWO

Let the lower body rotate towards the right, letting the left foot go on its side slightly. Allow the left hip to drop into a stretch. Return to the preparatory position, then repeat the stretch on the other side.

KEY

- •-- *Joints*
- ○— *Muscles*
- ● Shortening with tension
- ● Lengthening with tension
- ● Lengthening without tension
- ● Held muscles without motion

Chest and arms

The **left pectorals** and **biceps** are stretched as the arm presses into the floor and the trunk rotates away. The **right shoulder** and **elbow extensors** engage to control the rotation.

133

HALF-KNEEL HIP FLEXOR STRETCH

This exercise is great for stretching the anterior hip, including the quad and hip flexor. The half-kneel position with both legs bent makes the stretch easy to achieve, due to shorter levers.

This stretch allows for relief of tension caused by excessively pushing the hip into extension. Using the breath and contraction in the glutes, the hip flexors reciprocally undergo a stretch. Achieving the stretch without a large change in joint position may be a better option for those who have range of motion limitations or a labral tear – an injury to the tissue that holds the ball-and-socket parts of the hip together.

KEY
- •-- *Joints*
- ○— *Muscles*
- ● Shortening with tension
- ● Lengthening with tension
- ○ Lengthening without tension
- ● Held muscles without motion

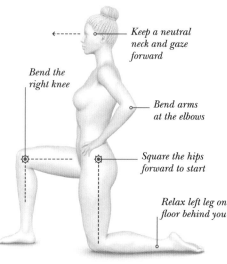

Keep a neutral neck and gaze forward

Bend the right knee

Bend arms at the elbows

Square the hips forward to start

Relax left leg on floor behind you

PREPARATORY STAGE
Begin in a half-kneeling position with your left knee bent on the floor and your right knee bent in front, right foot flat on the floor. Keep your spine neutral and your gaze forward.

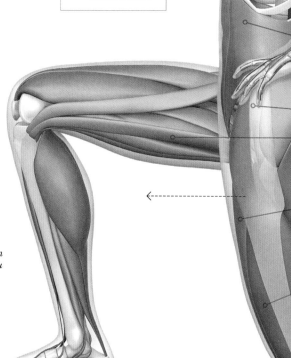

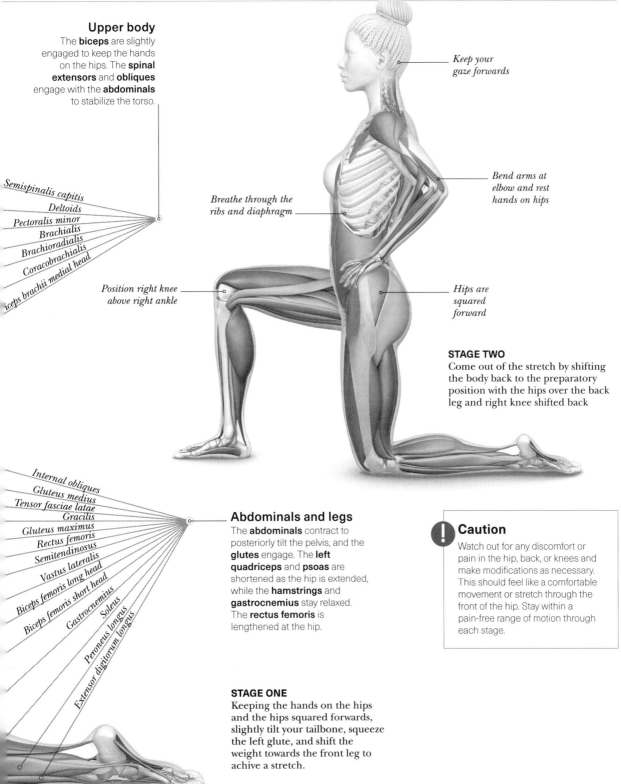

Upper body

The **biceps** are slightly engaged to keep the hands on the hips. The **spinal extensors** and **obliques** engage with the **abdominals** to stabilize the torso.

Semispinalis capitis
Deltoids
Pectoralis minor
Brachialis
Brachioradialis
Coracobrachialis
Biceps brachii medial head

Breathe through the ribs and diaphragm

Position right knee above right ankle

Keep your gaze forwards

Bend arms at elbow and rest hands on hips

Hips are squared forward

STAGE TWO
Come out of the stretch by shifting the body back to the preparatory position with the hips over the back leg and right knee shifted back

Internal obliques
Gluteus medius
Tensor fasciae latae
Gracilis
Gluteus maximus
Rectus femoris
Semitendinosus
Vastus lateralis
Biceps femoris long head
Biceps femoris short head
Gastrocnemius
Soleus
Peroneus longus
Extensor digitorum longus

Abdominals and legs

The **abdominals** contract to posteriorly tilt the pelvis, and the **glutes** engage. The **left quadriceps** and **psoas** are shortened as the hip is extended, while the **hamstrings** and **gastrocnemius** stay relaxed. The **rectus femoris** is lengthened at the hip.

! Caution
Watch out for any discomfort or pain in the hip, back, or knees and make modifications as necessary. This should feel like a comfortable movement or stretch through the front of the hip. Stay within a pain-free range of motion through each stage.

STAGE ONE
Keeping the hands on the hips and the hips squared forwards, slightly tilt your tailbone, squeeze the left glute, and shift the weight towards the front leg to achive a stretch.

» VARIATIONS

Hip flexor mobility can affect hip extension. Standing variations of the Half-kneel Hip Flexor Stretch are a good alternative, and transfer into activities such as climbing stairs.

STANDING HIP FLEXOR STRETCH

This stretch is a great alternative for those who have trouble performing the half-kneeling version of this exercise (see p.134). It utilizes pelvic position and the glute to provide a stretch to the hip flexors and can be done to help reduce muscle tension and encourage flexibility.

KEY
● Primary target muscle
● Secondary target muscle

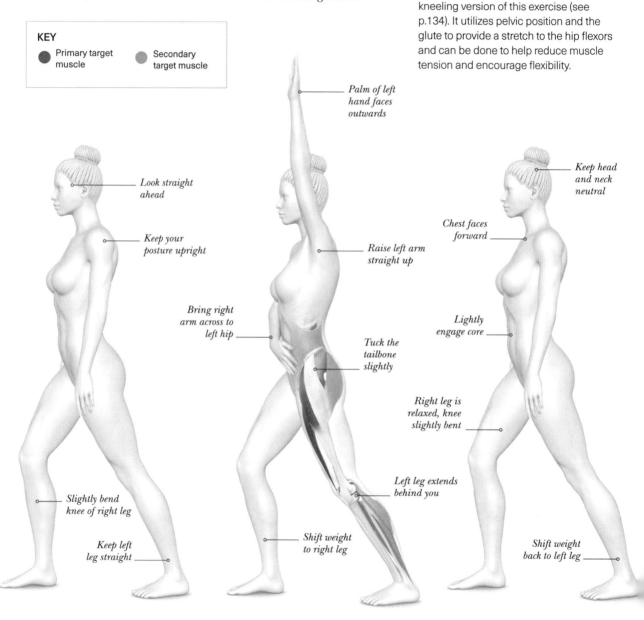

Look straight ahead

Keep your posture upright

Bring right arm across to left hip

Slightly bend knee of right leg

Keep left leg straight

Palm of left hand faces outwards

Raise left arm straight up

Tuck the tailbone slightly

Left leg extends behind you

Shift weight to right leg

Keep head and neck neutral

Chest faces forward

Lightly engage core

Right leg is relaxed, knee slightly bent

Shift weight back to left leg

PREPARATORY STAGE
Begin in a split stance with your right leg forward and slightly bent. Keep your left leg back and straight.

STAGE ONE
Tuck the tailbone slightly and shift your body weight to the front leg while reaching upwards with the left arm. At the same time, bring the right arm across the hips.

STAGE TWO
Lower the left arm, bring the right arm back by your side, and shift your weight forward again.

CHAIR/ELEVATED HIP FLEXOR STRETCH

This variation is perfect for those with limited hip extension range of motion. Using a chair allows the opposite hip to be flexed, making it easier to achieve a good stretch in the hip flexor.

Caution
Be mindful of any discomfort deep in the hip. Structural variations or changes in this region may affect available hip joint range of motion. Modify by not moving the stance leg into as much extension.

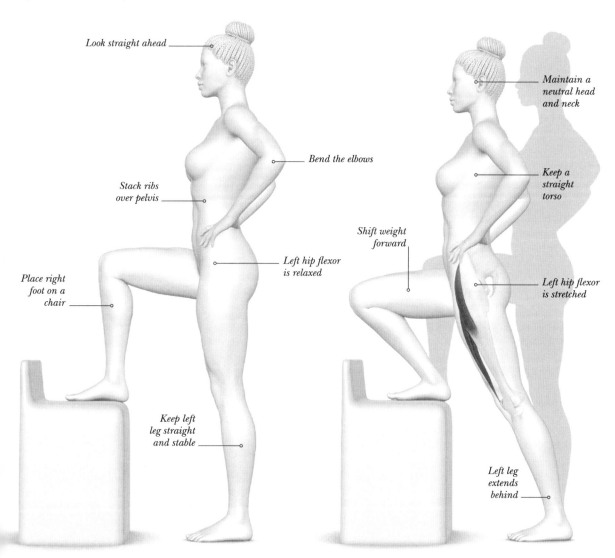

Look straight ahead

Bend the elbows

Stack ribs over pelvis

Left hip flexor is relaxed

Place right foot on a chair

Keep left leg straight and stable

Maintain a neutral head and neck

Keep a straight torso

Shift weight forward

Left hip flexor is stretched

Left leg extends behind

PREPARATORY STAGE

STAGE ONE

PREPARATORY STAGE
Place the right foot on a chair or bench to achieve a split stance with the front leg elevated.

STAGE ONE
Press the back heel into the floor to fully extend the back leg, while slightly shifting the body forward so you feel a stretch in the left hip flexor.

STAGE TWO
Shift your body weight back to come out of the stretch.

137

PIGEON STRETCH

The hip rotators can be stretched a variety of ways. The seated Pigeon Stretch allows for the intensity of the stretch to be controlled by how much weight is allowed through it.

It's not uncommon for this area to feel tight due to high volumes of lower body exercise and rotational movements. Adjust the angle of the target hip and gently sink further into the pose to achieve the stretch. You should feel it in the posterior hip and glute.

KEY

●-- *Joints*

○— *Muscles*

● Shortening with tension

● Lengthening with tension

● Lengthening without tension

● Held muscles without motion

Front hip and leg
The **right adductors** are engaged, and the **right glute** and **hip rotators** lengthen under tension. The **left hip flexors** lengthen as the **quadriceps** and **hip extensors** extend the leg.

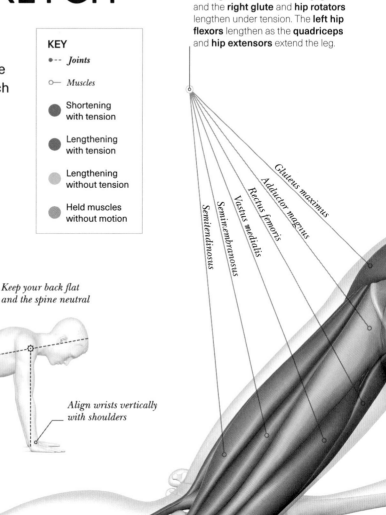

Gluteus maximus

Adductor magnus

Rectus femoris

Vastus medialis

Semimembranosus

Semitendinosus

PREPARATORY STAGE
Begin in the four-point kneeling position with your elbows straight and hands below your shoulders. Align your knees under your hips.

Keep your back flat and the spine neutral

Align wrists vertically with shoulders

Align knees vertically with hips

STAGE TWO
Lower down onto the forearms to hold the stretch to the desired depth. Adjust the angle of the stretch by moving the knee higher or lower to change the hip flexion angle. Then extend the arms and uncross your leg to repeat the other side.

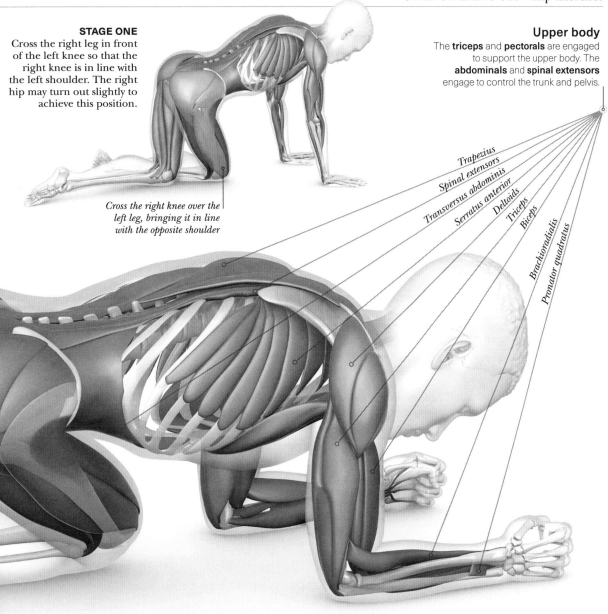

STAGE ONE
Cross the right leg in front of the left knee so that the right knee is in line with the left shoulder. The right hip may turn out slightly to achieve this position.

Cross the right knee over the left leg, bringing it in line with the opposite shoulder

Upper body
The **triceps** and **pectorals** are engaged to support the upper body. The **abdominals** and **spinal extensors** engage to control the trunk and pelvis.

Trapezius
Spinal extensors
Transversus abdominis
Serratus anterior
Deltoids
Triceps
Biceps
Brachioradialis
Pronator quadratus

VARIATION: SEATED

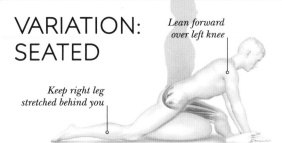

Lean forward over left knee

Keep right leg stretched behind you

PREPARATORY STAGE
Begin seated on a block or a pillow with the right leg extended behind you and the left leg externally rotated. Balance by placing your fingertips lightly on the floor either side of the bent leg, or if using a pillow, flat on the pillow. If you can't reach the floor, place a yoga block under each hand.

STAGE ONE
Move your hands in front of you and lean forward with hands on the floor. Fold over the left hip to achieve the complete stretch.

STAGE TWO
Bring the torso upright again, letting the hands rest either side of your body as in the preparatory pose.

WORLD'S GREATEST STRETCH

This dynamic, active stretch lives up to its name – stretching the hips, ankles, and thoracic spine. It is a favourite for many athletes and active people as it strengthens and lengthens the body through the movement.

The World's Greatest Stretch is a three-part stretch that targets multiple areas in a single sequence. The lunge forward emphasizes hip mobility while the elbow-to-floor and rotation emphasizes thoracic mobility. It requires coordination and body control and can serve as an excellent dynamic warmup for any workout, such as weight lifting or running, and is especially great for multiplanar sports like soccer, baseball, or volleyball.

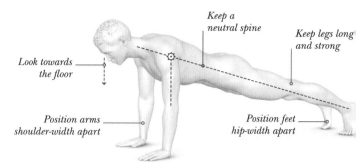

Look towards the floor

Keep a neutral spine

Keep legs long and strong

Position arms shoulder-width apart

Position feet hip-width apart

PREPARATORY STAGE
Begin in a high plank position, resting on your hands and toes with a neutral spine and hands roughly shoulder-width apart.

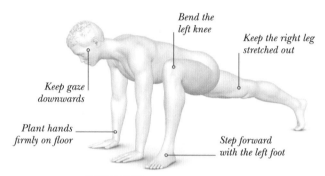

Bend the left knee

Keep the right leg stretched out

Keep gaze downwards

Plant hands firmly on floor

Step forward with the left foot

STAGE ONE
Step forward to bring the left foot next to the left hand, assuming a lunge stance, your left foot placed outside your left hand.

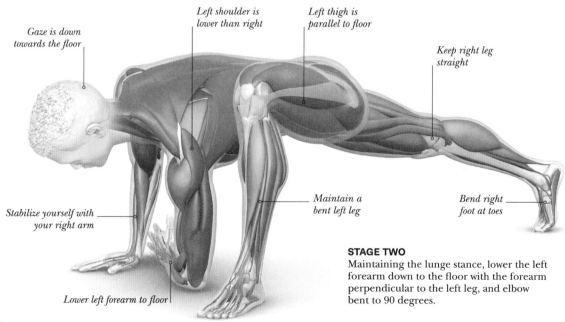

Gaze is down towards the floor

Left shoulder is lower than right

Left thigh is parallel to floor

Keep right leg straight

Stabilize yourself with your right arm

Maintain a bent left leg

Bend right foot at toes

Lower left forearm to floor

STAGE TWO
Maintaining the lunge stance, lower the left forearm down to the floor with the forearm perpendicular to the left leg, and elbow bent to 90 degrees.

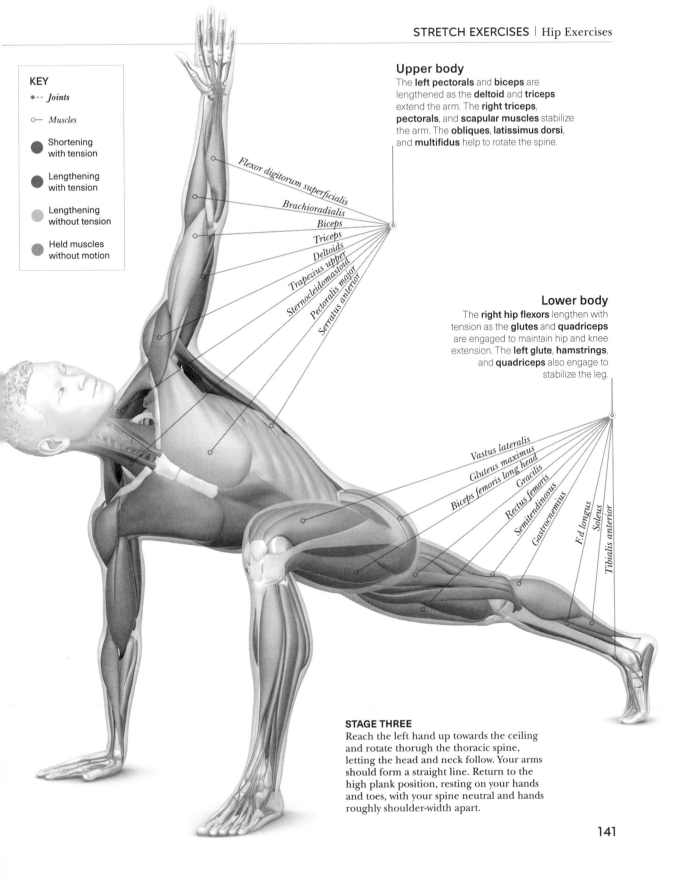

KEY

●-- *Joints*

○— *Muscles*

● Shortening with tension

● Lengthening with tension

○ Lengthening without tension

● Held muscles without motion

Flexor digitorum superficialis

Brachioradialis

Biceps

Triceps

Deltoids

Trapezius upper

Sternocleidomastoid

Pectoralis major

Serratus anterior

Upper body

The **left pectorals** and **biceps** are lengthened as the **deltoid** and **triceps** extend the arm. The **right triceps**, **pectorals**, and **scapular muscles** stabilize the arm. The **obliques**, **latissimus dorsi**, and **multifidus** help to rotate the spine.

Lower body

The **right hip flexors** lengthen with tension as the **glutes** and **quadriceps** are engaged to maintain hip and knee extension. The **left glute**, **hamstrings**, and **quadriceps** also engage to stabilize the leg.

Vastus lateralis

Gluteus maximus

Biceps femoris long head

Gracilis

Rectus femoris

Semitendinosus

Gastrocnemius

F.d longus

Soleus

Tibialis anterior

STAGE THREE

Reach the left hand up towards the ceiling and rotate thorugh the thoracic spine, letting the head and neck follow. Your arms should form a straight line. Return to the high plank position, resting on your hands and toes, with your spine neutral and hands roughly shoulder-width apart.

141

PANCAKE STRETCH

The ultimate goal of this exercise is to achieve a completely flat posture – like a pancake – which will take practice. It provides an active stretch for the hips, hamstrings, lower back, and adductors (inner thighs).

The Pancake Stretch, which involves a forward fold of the trunk, is performed on the floor as part of a lower body stretch routine and is particularly helpful for dancers. Use the hands to support how far you can comfortably lower into the stretch, and position the legs as wide as you can tolerate. With time and practice, you will be able to increase the depth of your stretch. Try the seated variation if you have difficulty stretching on the floor.

66 99

The adductor muscle group spans the medial part of the thigh and primarily adducts the leg, but also assists with other motions.

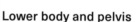

Gluteus maximus
Gluteus medius
Tensor fasciae latae
Rectus femoris
Vastus lateralis
Biceps femoris long head

Lower body and pelvis
The **hip flexors** contract to lower the torso. The **adductors, semitendinosus, semimembranosus, biceps femoris,** and **calves** are lengthened as the hips flex while abducted with knee extension and ankle dorsiflexion.

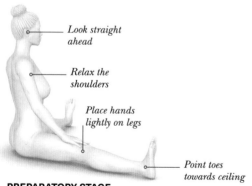

Look straight ahead

Relax the shoulders

Place hands lightly on legs

Point toes towards ceiling

PREPARATORY STAGE
Begin seated on the floor with legs wide in a "V" shape and hands resting lightly on your legs.

Caution
This should feel like a comfortable movement through the inner thighs. Gently increase intensity of this stretch and be sure to modify if you feel any discomfort.

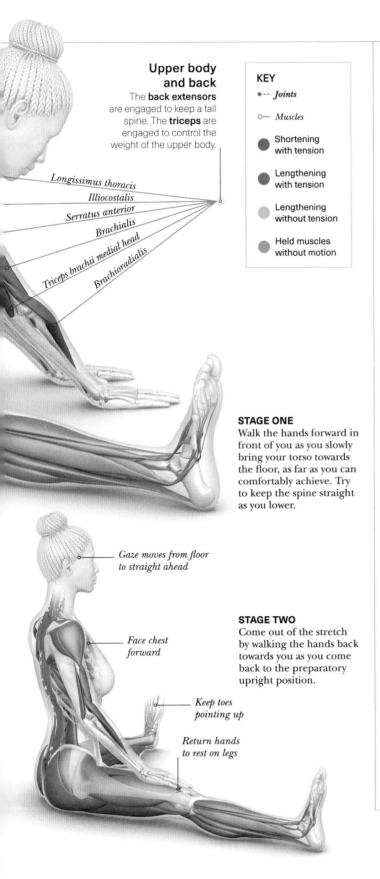

Upper body and back

The **back extensors** are engaged to keep a tall spine. The **triceps** are engaged to control the weight of the upper body.

Longissimus thoracis
Illiocostalis
Serratus anterior
Brachialis
Triceps brachii medial head
Brachioradialis

KEY

•-- *Joints*

○— *Muscles*

● Shortening with tension

● Lengthening with tension

○ Lengthening without tension

● Held muscles without motion

STAGE ONE
Walk the hands forward in front of you as you slowly bring your torso towards the floor, as far as you can comfortably achieve. Try to keep the spine straight as you lower.

Gaze moves from floor to straight ahead

Face chest forward

STAGE TWO
Come out of the stretch by walking the hands back towards you as you come back to the preparatory upright position.

Keep toes pointing up

Return hands to rest on legs

VARIATION: SEATED

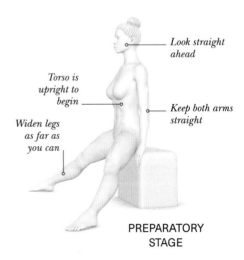

Look straight ahead

Torso is upright to begin

Keep both arms straight

Widen legs as far as you can

PREPARATORY STAGE

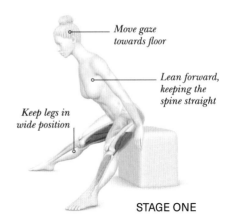

Move gaze towards floor

Lean forward, keeping the spine straight

Keep legs in wide position

STAGE ONE

PREPARATORY STAGE
Begin seated on a bench with the legs as wide as they comfortably can be in a "V" shape, feet relaxed, and hands holding the bench.

STAGE ONE
Keeping a straight back, lean forward, hinging at the hips to achieve the stretch in the hamstrings and adductors.

STAGE TWO
Maintaining a straight back, return to the preparatory stage.

HAPPY BABY POSE

When you are in the Happy Baby Pose, lying on the floor and holding your feet, you resemble a baby happily lying on its back. This gentle, opening pose stretches the hips and ankles, relaxes the pelvic floor, and can reduce tension in the lower back and hips.

By bringing the knees towards the chest, opening the hips, and focussing on breathing through the ribs and diaphragm, the pelvic floor is able to relax. If holding the feet is challenging, you may hold the ankles or shins instead. The gentle rock from side to side is optional, but can provide additional relaxation.

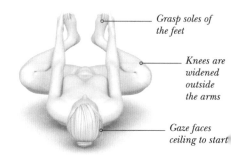

Grasp soles of the feet

Knees are widened outside the arms

Gaze faces ceiling to start

PREPARATORY STAGE
Begin lying on the floor on your back. Bring in your knees towards your chest and grasp the outsides of the feet.

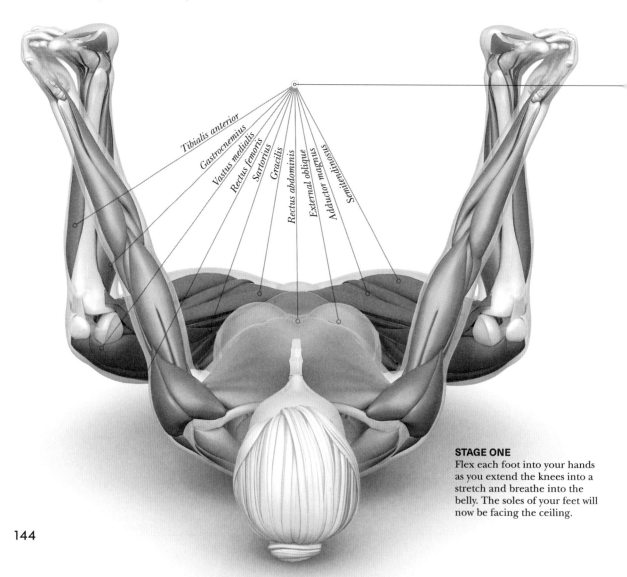

Tibialis anterior

Gastrocnemius

Vastus medialis

Rectus femoris

Sartorius

Gracilis

Rectus abdominis

External oblique

Adductor magnus

Semitendinosus

STAGE ONE
Flex each foot into your hands as you extend the knees into a stretch and breathe into the belly. The soles of your feet will now be facing the ceiling.

VARIATION: SINGLE LEG

PREPARATORY STAGE
Begin lying flat on the floor. Grasp the outside of the left foot with your left hand and bring the left knee towards the chest, keeping the right leg extended and relaxed.

STAGE ONE
Flex the left foot into the hand as you extend the knee into a stretch and breathe into the belly, leaving the right leg extended in front of you.

STAGE TWO
Gently rock from side to side while maintaining the stretch in the left leg, and using the grounded right hand to help control the movement.

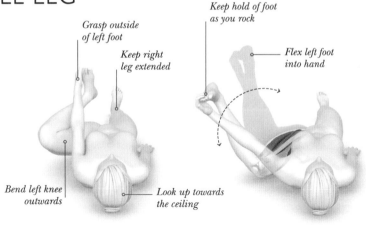

Grasp outside of left foot

Keep right leg extended

Keep hold of foot as you rock

Flex left foot into hand

Bend left knee outwards

Look up towards the ceiling

PREPARATORY STAGE

STAGE ONE / TWO

Pelvis and legs
The chest is aimed forward while the hands pull the legs into a stretch. The **hip adductors**, **hamstrings**, and **calves** are stretched during this position. The **ankles** are dorsiflexed and the **hips** are flexed and abducted.

 Caution
Be mindful of positioning in the Happy Baby Pose if you have hip or knee pain. This stretch is not recommended after the first trimester during pregnancy.

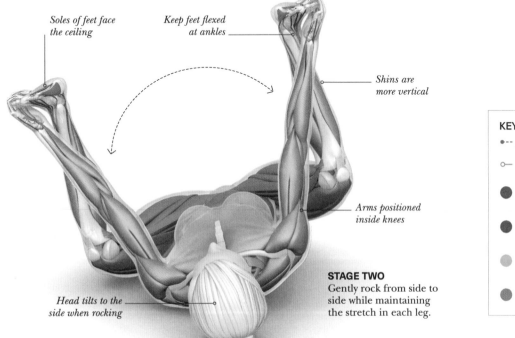

Soles of feet face the ceiling

Keep feet flexed at ankles

Shins are more vertical

Arms positioned inside knees

Head tilts to the side when rocking

STAGE TWO
Gently rock from side to side while maintaining the stretch in each leg.

KEY
- ●--- *Joints*
- ○— *Muscles*
- ● Shortening with tension
- ● Lengthening with tension
- ● Lengthening without tension
- ● Held muscles without motion

145

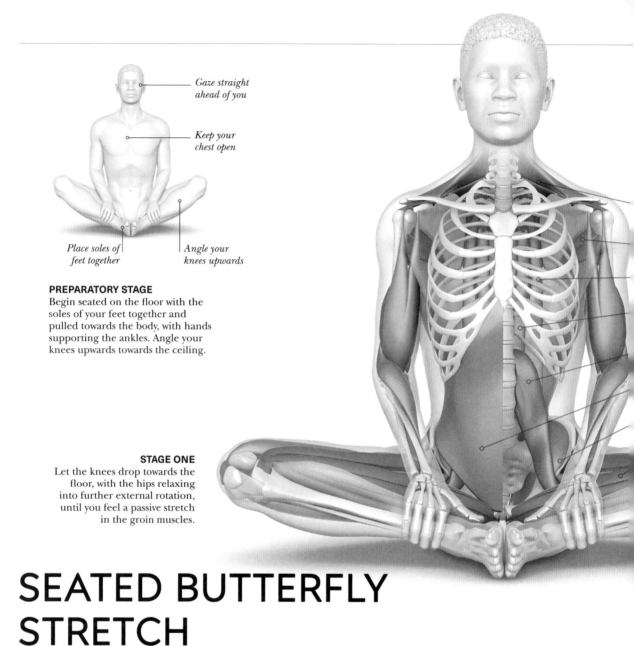

Gaze straight
ahead of you

Keep your
chest open

Place soles of
feet together

Angle your
knees upwards

PREPARATORY STAGE
Begin seated on the floor with the
soles of your feet together and
pulled towards the body, with hands
supporting the ankles. Angle your
knees upwards towards the ceiling.

STAGE ONE
Let the knees drop towards the
floor, with the hips relaxing
into further external rotation,
until you feel a passive stretch
in the groin muscles.

SEATED BUTTERFLY STRETCH

This seated exercise is great for stretching the hips and adductors (inner thighs), as
it stretches into abduction and external rotation. Reducing tension in the adductors
may be helpful for managing hip and knee pain.

The Butterfly Stretch, popular in yoga, is a
foundational stretch used in many fitness classes. You
can add a forward fold to intensify the stretch, or
practise addressing the groin and inner thigh as the
hips externally rotate with the soles of the feet
together, using the help of gravity or added external
pressure. If you can't bring the ankles that far in, go
as far as you can. If the stretch is too intense, place
pillows under the knees to reduce the range of
motion of the stretch.

Trunk and lower body

The **back extensors** are engaged to maintain an upright spine. The **pectineus**, **adductor longus**, and **adductor brevis** are the primary adductors lengthened without tension.

Sternocleidomastoid
Teres minor
Illiocostalis
Longissimus thoracis
Psoas major
Transversus abdominis
Iliacus
Gracilis
Sartorius
Vastus medialis

VARIATION: SUPINE

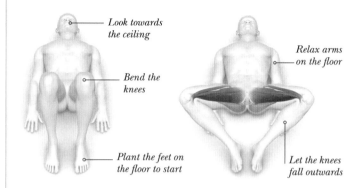

Look towards the ceiling

Bend the knees

Plant the feet on the floor to start

Relax arms on the floor

Let the knees fall outwards

PREPARATORY STAGE

Begin lying on your back on the floor with your knees bent, feet relaxed, and arms stretched out by your sides.

STAGE ONE

Let the knees fall outwards slowly into a stretch for as long as desired. Return the knees to the centre to come out of the stretch.

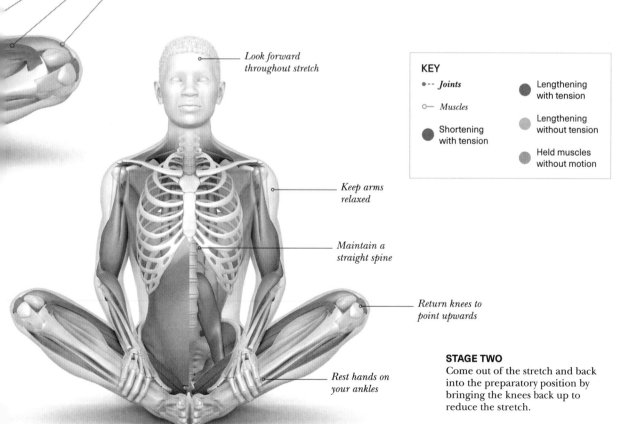

Look forward throughout stretch

Keep arms relaxed

Maintain a straight spine

Return knees to point upwards

Rest hands on your ankles

KEY

•-- *Joints*

o— *Muscles*

● Shortening with tension

● Lengthening with tension

● Lengthening without tension

● Held muscles without motion

STAGE TWO

Come out of the stretch and back into the preparatory position by bringing the knees back up to reduce the stretch.

STANDING HIP CIRCLES

These hip-controlled articular rotations (CARs), allow you to actively move through your entire available joint mobility. They promote active mobility in the hip joint, while also improving balance and stability on the standing leg. See variations (p.150) for kneeling and lying versions.

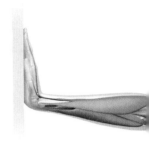

Hip Circles offer mobility, strength, and coordination and can be used as a daily movement exercise, as part of a hip or lower body programme, and as a warmup. It's important to explore and understand your available hip mobility so that you are aware of your range of motion. Understanding and practising hip circles can serve as a good precursor to additional strength training for certain sports to increase joint resilience.

> **! Caution**
>
> Watch out for any discomfort or pain in the hip, back, or knees. Non-painful noises can be normal with joints. If you have any pinching or sharp pain, avoid pushing through it – stay within a pain-free range of motion through each stage.

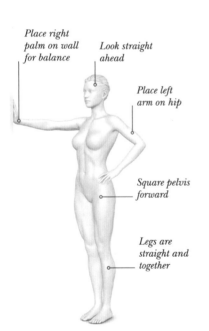

Place right palm on wall for balance

Look straight ahead

Place left arm on hip

Square pelvis forward

Legs are straight and together

PREPARATORY STAGE
Begin standing with weight evenly distributed through each leg. Place your right hand on a wall in preparation for balance assistance as you move to stage 1.

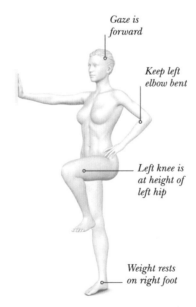

Gaze is forward

Keep left elbow bent

Left knee is at height of left hip

Weight rests on right foot

STAGE ONE
Shift your weight onto the right leg and stay tall. Drive the left knee up and forward as far as you comfortably can.

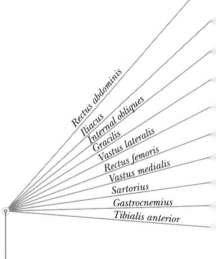

Rectus abdominis
Iliacus
Internal obliques
Gracilis
Vastus lateralis
Rectus femoris
Vastus medialis
Sartorius
Gastrocnemius
Tibialis anterior

Standing leg and abdomen
The **abdominals**, **tensor fasciae latae**, and **glutes** are engaged to stabilize the hip. The **quadriceps** are engaged to maintain knee extension. The **gastrocnemius**, **tibialis anterior**, and other lower leg muscles help stabilize the foot and ankle.

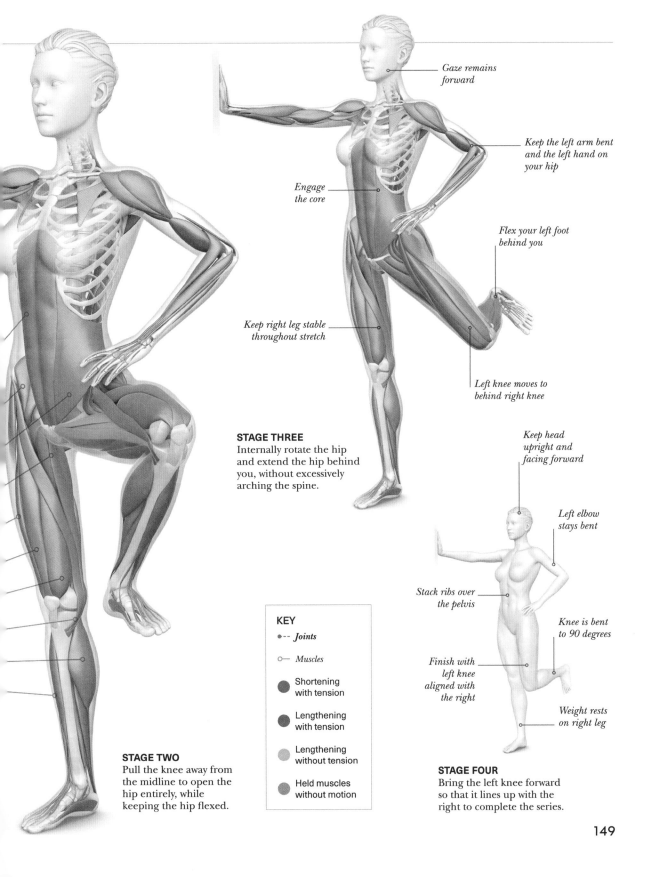

Gaze remains
forward

Keep the left arm bent
and the left hand on
your hip

Engage
the core

Flex your left foot
behind you

Keep right leg stable
throughout stretch

Left knee moves to
behind right knee

STAGE THREE
Internally rotate the hip
and extend the hip behind
you, without excessively
arching the spine.

Keep head
upright and
facing forward

Left elbow
stays bent

Stack ribs over
the pelvis

Knee is bent
to 90 degrees

Finish with
left knee
aligned with
the right

Weight rests
on right leg

STAGE TWO
Pull the knee away from
the midline to open the
hip entirely, while
keeping the hip flexed.

STAGE FOUR
Bring the left knee forward
so that it lines up with the
right to complete the series.

» VARIATIONS

You can practise hip circles in many positions, each suitable for different levels of skill or to emphasize various muscular demands.

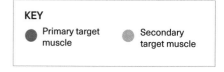
QUADRUPED HIP CIRCLE

The quadruped variation for the hip circle provides the challenge of moving against gravity. It is less intense than the standing version and a better option for sensitive hips with limited strength.

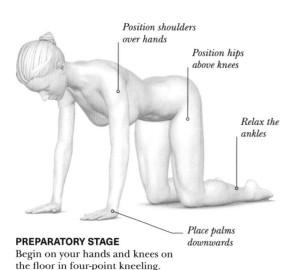

Position shoulders over hands

Position hips above knees

Relax the ankles

Place palms downwards

PREPARATORY STAGE
Begin on your hands and knees on the floor in four-point kneeling.

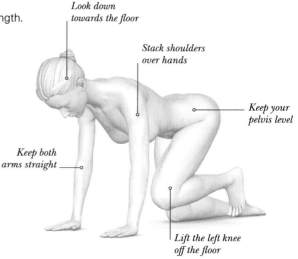

Look down towards the floor

Stack shoulders over hands

Keep your pelvis level

Keep both arms straight

Lift the left knee off the floor

STAGE ONE
Lift the left knee and flex the left hip towards the left elbow, while maintaining a level pelvis and keeping the lumbar spine stable.

SIDELYING HIP CIRCLE

This sidelying variation involves moving against gravity in the frontal plane. It can be a comfortable alternative for those who can't assume a four-point position, or perform the standing variation. It may also be a better option if you have sensitive or weak hips.

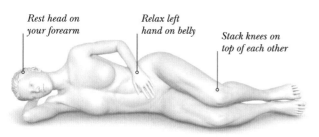

Rest head on your forearm

Relax left hand on belly

Stack knees on top of each other

Open left leg up and out

Keep chest facing forwards

Flex left leg towards chest

PREPARATORY STAGE
Begin lying on your right side with the knees and ankles stacked and the hips flexed. Rest your head on your right forearm.

STAGE ONE
Flex the left hip towards the chest while maintaining a square pelvis and minimizing movement at the lumbar spine.

STAGE TWO
Pull the knee away from the midline to open the hip. Try to avoid any rocking of the trunk or hips when you perform this movement.

66 99

Choose a variation that places a suitable level of demand on the core and pelvis.

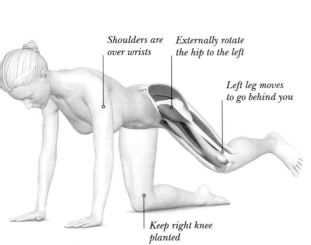

Shoulders are over wrists

Externally rotate the hip to the left

Left leg moves to go behind you

Keep right knee planted

STAGE TWO
Pull the knee away from the midline to open the hip entirely to the left side, while maintaining the other three points of contact with the floor.

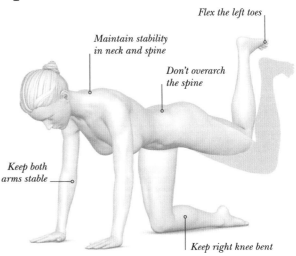

Flex the left toes

Maintain stability in neck and spine

Don't overarch the spine

Keep both arms stable

Keep right knee bent

STAGE THREE
Extend the left hip behind you then raise the leg so that so that the base of the foot faces the ceiling and knee is faces the floor.

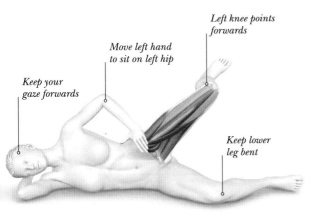

Left knee points forwards

Move left hand to sit on left hip

Keep your gaze forwards

Keep lower leg bent

STAGE THREE
Internally rotate the hip and pull it behind you without excessively arching the spine. You may place the left hand on the left hip so that body awareness will stop this from happening.

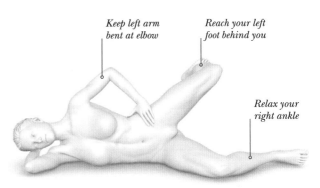

Keep left arm bent at elbow

Reach your left foot behind you

Relax your right ankle

STAGE FOUR
Extend the left hip fully so that the foot reaches back behind you, and the knee is pointed forward. Return to the preparatory stacked position.

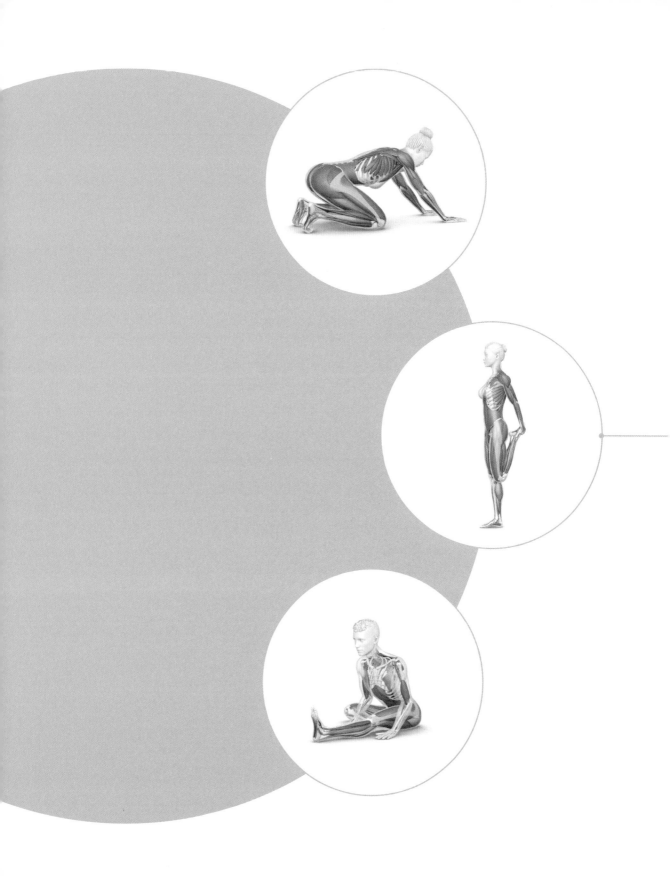

LEG AND FOOT EXERCISES

The leg plays a vital role in supporting body weight, facilitating movement, and maintaining balance. Stretching to retain an adequate range of motion in the knee, foot, and ankle joints allows for natural movement patterns like walking, and ease of functional tasks like stair climbing. Flexible, strong legs and feet also enhance performance when taking part in sports such as running and cycling.

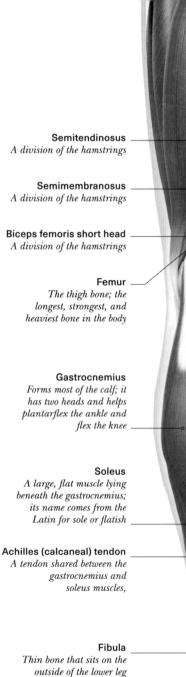

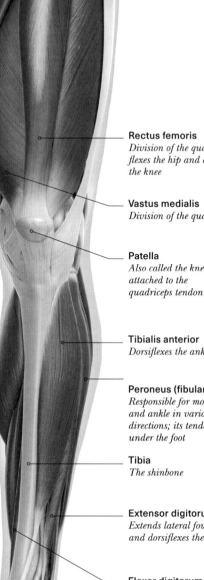

Semitendinosus
A division of the hamstrings

Semimembranosus
A division of the hamstrings

Biceps femoris short head
A division of the hamstrings

Femur
The thigh bone; the longest, strongest, and heaviest bone in the body

Gastrocnemius
Forms most of the calf; it has two heads and helps plantarflex the ankle and flex the knee

Soleus
A large, flat muscle lying beneath the gastrocnemius; its name comes from the Latin for sole or flatish

Achilles (calcaneal) tendon
A tendon shared between the gastrocnemius and soleus muscles,

Fibula
Thin bone that sits on the outside of the lower leg

Calcaneus
The heel bone

Rectus femoris
Division of the quads; flexes the hip and extends the knee

Vastus medialis
Division of the quadriceps

Patella
Also called the kneecap, attached to the quadriceps tendon

Tibialis anterior
Dorsiflexes the ankle

Peroneus (fibularis) longus
Responsible for moving the foot and ankle in various directions; its tendon wraps under the foot

Tibia
The shinbone

Extensor digitorum longus
Extends lateral four digits and dorsiflexes the ankle

Flexor digitorum longus
Flexes the second to fifth toes and helps plantarflexion of the ankle

Extensor hallucis longus
Flexes the big toe and helps plantarflexion of the ankle

POSTERIOR VIEW

ANTERIOR VIEW

LEG AND FOOT OVERVIEW

The major muscles of the lower leg, ankle, and foot include the calf muscles (gastrocnemius and soleus), the tibialis anterior, tibialis posterior, peroneal muscles, toe flexors, and intrinsic foot muscles. They contribute to movements such as plantarflexion, dorsiflexion, inversion, eversion, and toe movements.

The lower leg and foot muscles collaborate to help stabilize and propel the body forward. The calf muscles are crucial for everyday activities that require pushing off the ground, such as walking, running, and jumping. Other muscles like the tibialis anterior, peroneals, posterior tibialis, and flexor hallucis longus help to control the ankle and foot, and intrinsic foot muscles maintain arches, balance, and toe movements.

Flexibility exercises such as calf stretches enhance range of motion in this region, while strength training, targeting these muscle groups, improves stability, power, and endurance. Developing strong and flexible muscles in the leg and foot area help you perform everyday activities with ease, and reduce the risk of injury that can be sustained either in daily life or sports.

STANDING QUAD STRETCH

This simple stretch is very versatile – you can practise it anywhere, whether at home or out for a run or walk. It stretches the quadriceps, or quad muscle, which is located at the front of the thigh and is a knee extensor and hip flexor.

If you are unable to reach the ankle with your hand to perform this stretch, try using a strap around the foot. Place one hand against a wall or railing if you need help balancing. This stretch can form part of a lower body routine or be used as a daily stretch. In order to maximize the muscle pull, be careful not to let the knee drift forward, or the back to arch excessivly.

Caution

Slightly tuck the tailbone so the pelvis helps to resist compensatory tilting, resulting in lower back extension. Be mindful of any limitations in knee range of motion or pain that may hinder your ability to comfortably achieve this stretch.

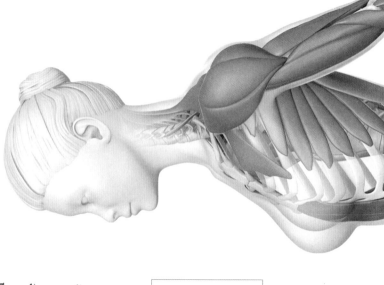

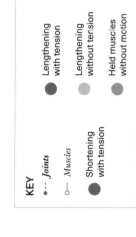

Look straight ahead of you

Relax arms by your sides to start

Legs are hip-width apart

Distribute weight evenly between both feet

PREPARATORY STAGE
Begin standing with feet hip-width apart and arms relaxed loosely by your sides.

KEY

- - - Joints
- o— Muscles

Shortening with tension

Lengthening with tension

Lengthening without tension

Held muscles without motion

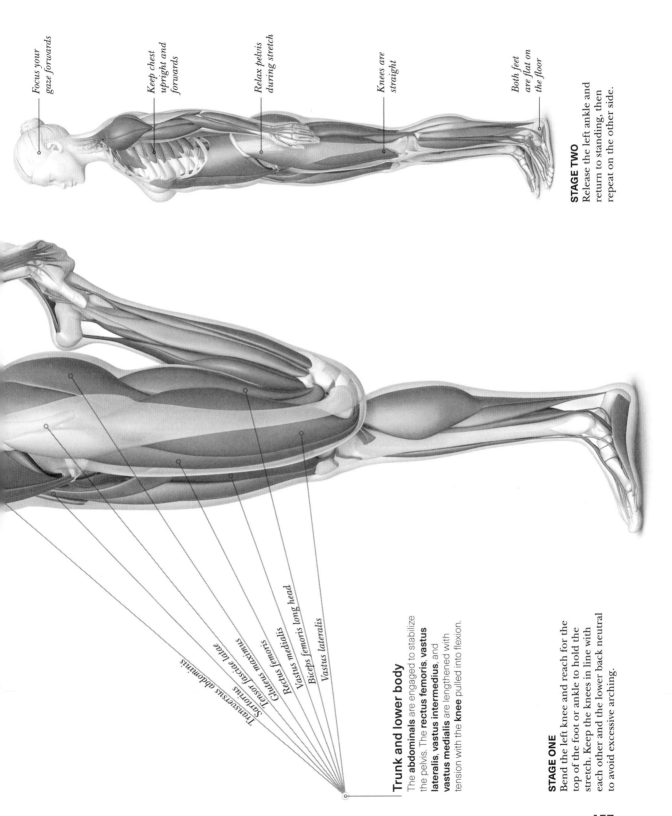

Focus your gaze forwards

Keep chest upright and forwards

Relax pelvis during stretch

Knees are straight

Both feet are flat on the floor

STAGE TWO
Release the left ankle and return to standing, then repeat on the other side.

Trunk and lower body

The **abdominals** are engaged to stabilize the pelvis. The **rectus femoris**, **vastus lateralis**, **vastus intermedius**, and **vastus medialis** are lengthened with tension with the **knee** pulled into flexion.

Transversus abdominis
Sartorius
Tensor fasciae latae
Gluteus maximus
Rectus medialis
Vastus medialis
Biceps femoris long head
Vastus lateralis

STAGE ONE
Bend the left knee and reach for the top of the foot or ankle to hold the stretch. Keep the knees in line with each other and the lower back neutral to avoid excessive arching.

157

» VARIATIONS

Different quadriceps stretches may be better suited for some people, depending on their available range of motion, skill level, or desired stretch intensity. Try the foot elevated variation for a gentle stretch, or choose the couch stretch for more intensity.

WITH FOOT ELEVATED

This variation is great for those who have limited knee flexion or are unable to reach the foot with the hand. If you need balance assistance, place the hands against a wall nearby.

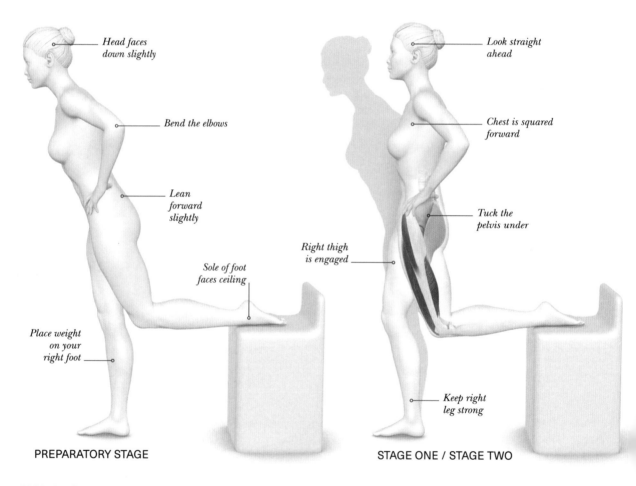

Head faces down slightly

Bend the elbows

Lean forward slightly

Sole of foot faces ceiling

Place weight on your right foot

PREPARATORY STAGE

Look straight ahead

Chest is squared forward

Tuck the pelvis under

Right thigh is engaged

Keep right leg strong

STAGE ONE / STAGE TWO

PREPARATORY STAGE
Begin standing with the top of the left foot propped behind you on a chair, sole of the foot facing up. Place your hands lightly on your hips, or if you need balance assistance, place your right hand on a wall beside you.

STAGE ONE
Slightly tuck the pelvis and straighten the trunk to achieve the stretch in the anterior left quad muscle.

STAGE TWO
Relax the pelvis and hinge forward to come out of the stretch, returning to the slightly bent-over preparatory position.

66 99

The more the knee is flexed, the greater the stretch will feel on your quadriceps.

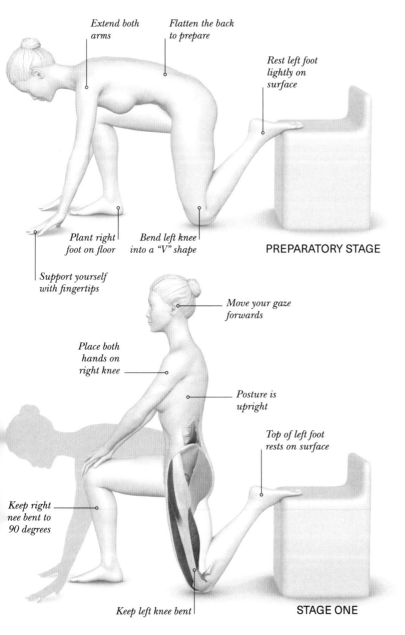

Extend both arms

Flatten the back to prepare

Rest left foot lightly on surface

Plant right foot on floor

Bend left knee into a "V" shape

Support yourself with fingertips

PREPARATORY STAGE

Move your gaze forwards

Place both hands on right knee

Posture is upright

Top of left foot rests on surface

Keep right knee bent to 90 degrees

Keep left knee bent

STAGE ONE

HALF-KNEEL COUCH STRETCH

This stretch targets the quad and hip flexors. To perform the stretch effectively, you need to be able to sustain pressure on the knee, as well as flexing it.

PREPARATORY STAGE
Begin in a half-kneel position, with the top of the left foot propped on a chair or couch. Lean forward with a flat back, supporting yourself with your fingertips on the floor in front of you.

STAGE ONE
Bring the trunk up and rest both arms on top of the right knee. Keep your tailbone slightly tucked under to avoid excessive lumbar extension.

STAGE TWO
Lower down to come out of the stretch, returning to the preparatory position, placing your fingertips on the floor to support you.

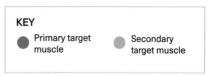

KEY

● Primary target muscle

● Secondary target muscle

STATIC HAMSTRING STRETCH

This classic stretch targets the hamstring muscle group. It can accompany a lower body programme or may be a helpful exercise for improving knee and hip mobility. You should feel the stretch at the back of the thigh.

The hamstrings originate at the pelvis and run behind the length of the femur, attaching below the knee. These muscles play a key role in hip extension and knee flexion. If your hamstrings are inflexible, you may experience limited knee extension efficiency and knee pain. Limited sciatic nerve mobility – the nerve that runs from the back of the pelvis and ends at the feet – may influence the hamstrings as well. Pair this stretch with strength training to improve strength and flexibility in this important muscle group.

> ❝❞
>
> *The hamstrings are comprised of three individual muscles: the semitendinosus, semimembranosus, and biceps femoris.*

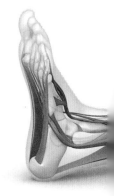

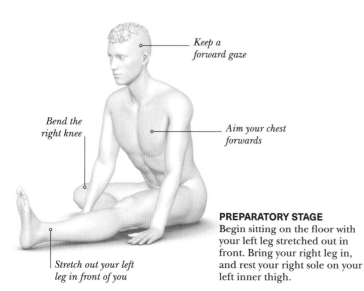

Keep a forward gaze

Bend the right knee

Aim your chest forwards

Stretch out your left leg in front of you

PREPARATORY STAGE
Begin sitting on the floor with your left leg stretched out in front. Bring your right leg in, and rest your right sole on your left inner thigh.

Lower body
The **hamstrings** are lengthened with tension with the **hip** flexed and **knee** extended. The **gastrocnemius** is lengthened without tension, while the **ankle** is dorsiflexed.

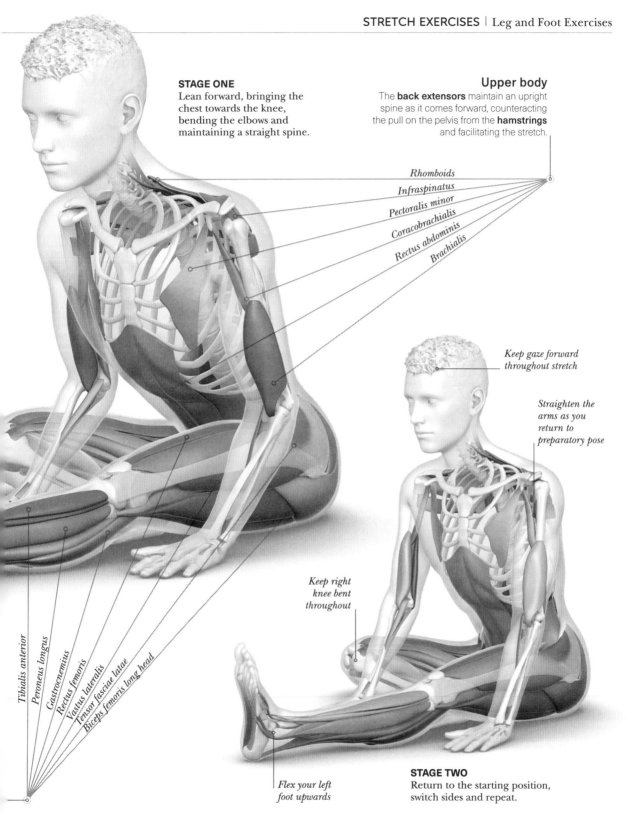

STAGE ONE
Lean forward, bringing the chest towards the knee, bending the elbows and maintaining a straight spine.

Upper body
The **back extensors** maintain an upright spine as it comes forward, counteracting the pull on the pelvis from the **hamstrings** and facilitating the stretch.

Rhomboids
Infraspinatus
Pectoralis minor
Coracobrachialis
Rectus abdominis
Brachialis

Keep gaze forward throughout stretch

Straighten the arms as you return to preparatory pose

Keep right knee bent throughout

Tibialis anterior
Peroneus longus
Gastrocnemius
Rectus femoris
Vastus lateralis
Tensor fasciae latae
Biceps femoris long head

Flex your left foot upwards

STAGE TWO
Return to the starting position, switch sides and repeat.

161

≫ VARIATIONS

These hamstring variations are less intense versions of the Static Hamstring Stretch (p.160). They are perfect for tension relief and promoting an increased range of motion.

Caution

If you feel any discomfort in the back or a burning sensation in the legs, try reducing the range of motion of the stretch or keeping the back flat. If symptoms persist, consult a professional for assessment.

SEATED HAMSTRING STRETCH

This seated variation of the Hamstring Stretch is a great way to stretch while working at a desk or sitting still for long periods of time. It can accompany a lower body programme or may be a helpful exercise for improving knee and hip mobility. You should feel a good stretch behind the thigh when you perform it.

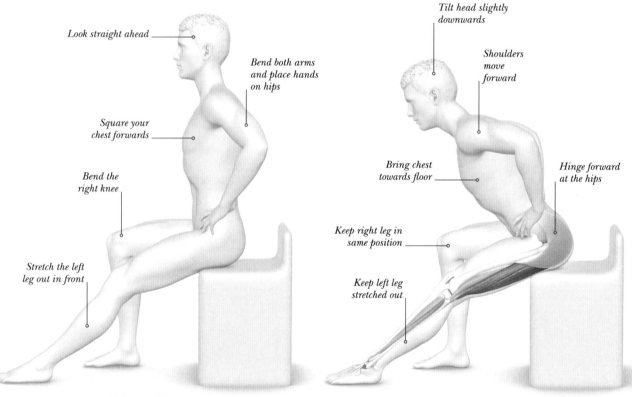

Look straight ahead

Bend both arms and place hands on hips

Square your chest forwards

Bend the right knee

Stretch the left leg out in front

PREPARATORY STAGE

Tilt head slightly downwards

Shoulders move forward

Bring chest towards floor

Hinge forward at the hips

Keep right leg in same position

Keep left leg stretched out

STAGE ONE

PREPARATORY STAGE
Sit on the edge of a chair with the left leg stretched out in front of the right and the left knee slightly bent. Place hands on your hips.

STAGE ONE
Lean forward, keeping the spine straight and hinging at the hips.

STAGE TWO
Return to the preparatory pose, bringing the back into an upright position.

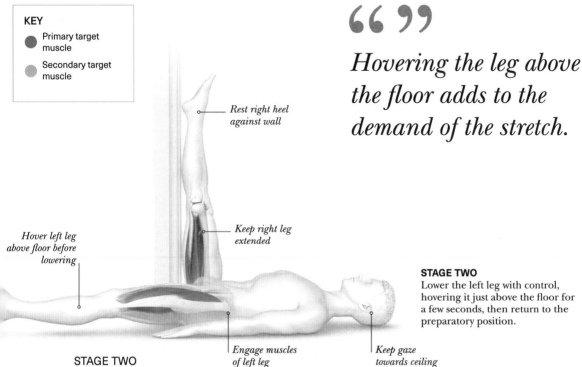

Flex the left foot

Rest right leg against doorway

Chest faces the ceiling

Left leg starts on floor

Rest arms by your sides

Look up towards ceiling

PREPARATORY STAGE / STAGE ONE

DYNAMIC HAMSTRING LOWERS

This hamstring stretch can be done as part of a warmup prior to exercise or sport. It involves holding a static stretch for the non-moving leg, while actively lowering and raising the opposite leg. This active movement of the hamstrings and hip flexors provides a dynamic stretch.

PREPARATORY STAGE
Begin lying on the floor with the right leg up against a doorway at a distance and angle sufficient to feel a mild stretch. Keep the left leg relaxed on the floor.

STAGE ONE
Bring the left leg up from the floor and past the right leg towards the chest. Flex your left foot.

KEY
- ● Primary target muscle
- ● Secondary target muscle

" "

Hovering the leg above the floor adds to the demand of the stretch.

Rest right heel against wall

Keep right leg extended

Hover left leg above floor before lowering

STAGE TWO
Lower the left leg with control, hovering it just above the floor for a few seconds, then return to the preparatory position.

Engage muscles of left leg

Keep gaze towards ceiling

STAGE TWO

163

GASTROCNEMIUS STEP STRETCH

The gastrocnemius is one of the largest muscles of the leg and consists of two heads that originate above the knee and make up the bulk of the calf muscle. It plays a significant role in propelling the body forward.

The gastrocnemius is a major ankle plantarflexor that assists with knee flexion. It also helps stabilize and control the ankle, particularly when walking. This stretch requires a small step, or you can use the bottom of a staircase. Use a hand rail for balance while you gradually lower into the stretch. For reduced intensity, keep one foot entirely on the step while the opposite heel drops below for a stretch. During the exercise, your forefeet should remain in contact with the step from the ball of the foot to the tips of the toes only. Keep your attention on the calves and Achilles tendon as you raise and drop the heels.

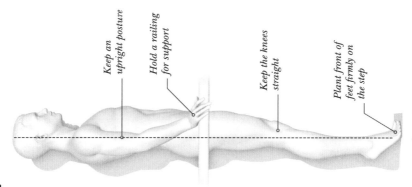

Keep an upright posture

Hold a railing for support

Keep the knees straight

Plant front of feet firmly on the step

PREPARATORY STAGE
Stand with feet under hips and with the balls of your feet on the step. Keep the weight evenly spread through the front of your feet and position feet parallel to the floor. Raise your heels as high as you can.

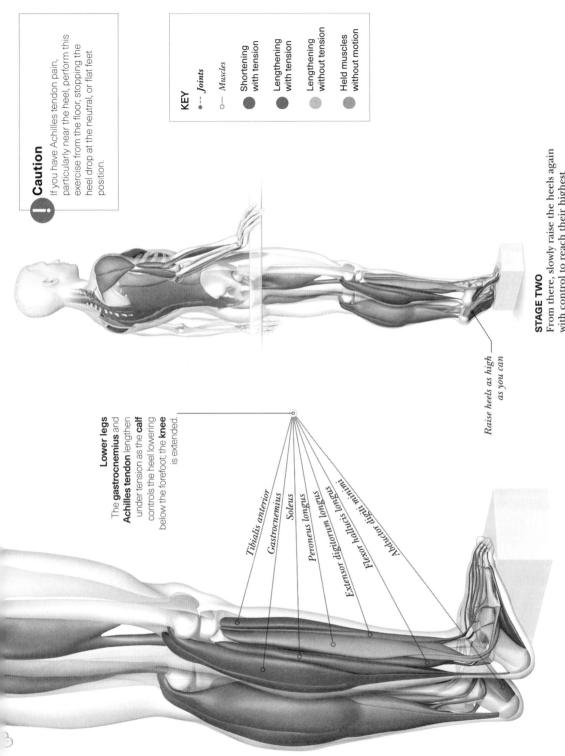

Caution

If you have Achilles tendon pain, particularly near the heel, perform this exercise from the floor, stopping the heel drop at the neutral, or flat feet position.

KEY

●--- *Joints*
○— *Muscles*

● Shortening with tension
● Lengthening with tension
● Lengthening without tension
● Held muscles without motion

Lower legs

The **gastrocnemius** and **Achilles tendon** lengthen under tension as the **calf** controls the heel lowering below the forefoot; the **knee** is extended.

Tibialis anterior
Gastrocnemius
Soleus
Peroneus longus
Extensor digitorum longus
Flexor hallucis minimi
Abductor digiti minimi

Raise heels as high as you can

STAGE TWO

From there, slowly raise the heels again with control to reach their highest position. Remember to maintain even weightbearing through the forefoot and minimize any toe gripping.

STAGE ONE

Slowly lower the heels, using the calf muscles, until you feel a stretch in the calf and Achilles tendon.

165

GASTROCNEMIUS WALL STRETCH

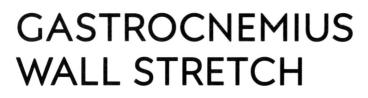

As an alternative to the step stretch (see p.164), the Gastrocnemius Wall Stretch is a simple weightbearing exercise that targets the gastrocnemius and Achilles tendon.

This stretch can be modified from a static to dynamic stretch by changing the hold times in stages one and two. It is a great stretch to maintain calf flexibility and ankle range of motion. This position is less intense than the step stretch and may be a better option for those who are can't tolerate actively lowering into the dorsiflexed position. Progress the stretch by pushing the heel down more and taking up more weight on the stance leg, or maintaining a single position for longer.

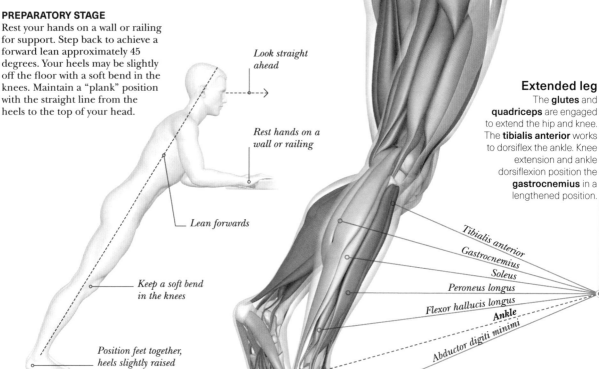

PREPARATORY STAGE
Rest your hands on a wall or railing for support. Step back to achieve a forward lean approximately 45 degrees. Your heels may be slightly off the floor with a soft bend in the knees. Maintain a "plank" position with the straight line from the heels to the top of your head.

Look straight ahead

Rest hands on a wall or railing

Lean forwards

Keep a soft bend in the knees

Position feet together, heels slightly raised

Extended leg
The **glutes** and **quadriceps** are engaged to extend the hip and knee. The **tibialis anterior** works to dorsiflex the ankle. Knee extension and ankle dorsiflexion position the **gastrocnemius** in a lengthened position.

Tibialis anterior
Gastrocnemius
Soleus
Peroneus longus
Flexor hallucis longus
Ankle
Abductor digiti minimi

166

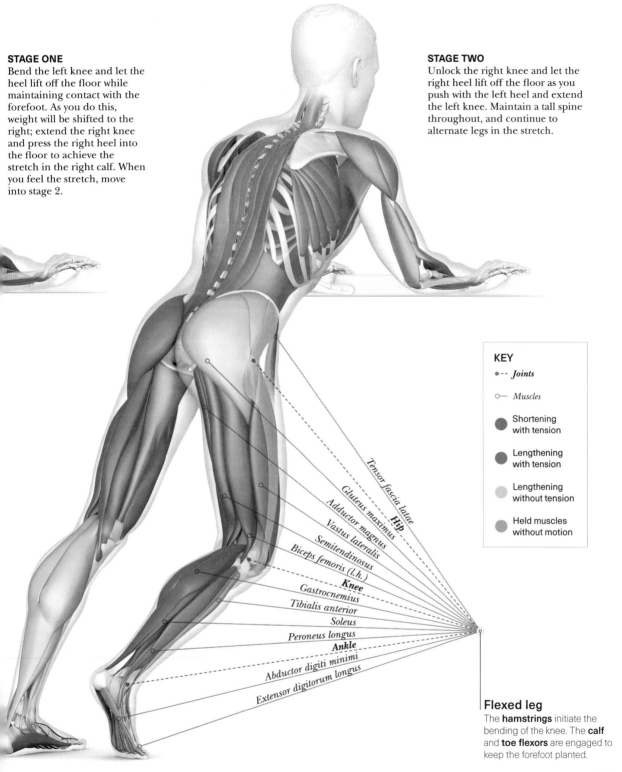

STAGE ONE
Bend the left knee and let the heel lift off the floor while maintaining contact with the forefoot. As you do this, weight will be shifted to the right; extend the right knee and press the right heel into the floor to achieve the stretch in the right calf. When you feel the stretch, move into stage 2.

STAGE TWO
Unlock the right knee and let the right heel lift off the floor as you push with the left heel and extend the left knee. Maintain a tall spine throughout, and continue to alternate legs in the stretch.

KEY

- ●-- *Joints*
- ○— *Muscles*
- ● Shortening with tension
- ● Lengthening with tension
- ● Lengthening without tension
- ● Held muscles without motion

Tensor fascia latae
Hip
Gluteus maximus
Adductor magnus
Vastus lateralis
Semitendinosus
Biceps femoris (l.h.)
Knee
Gastrocnemius
Tibialis anterior
Soleus
Peroneus longus
Ankle
Abductor digiti minimi
Extensor digitorum longus

Flexed leg
The **hamstrings** initiate the bending of the knee. The **calf** and **toe flexors** are engaged to keep the forefoot planted.

167

» VARIATIONS

Various calf and ankle stretches utilize different amounts of body weight and different joint angles. These stretches will help you to choose the best option for your desired physical activity goals and current ability.

BENT-KNEE CALF STRETCH

To stretch the lower of the two main calf muscles, the soleus, you must add a slight knee bend to the classic calf stretch. The Bent-knee Calf Stretch can supplement a standing calf stretch and helps to maintain ankle mobility and calf flexibility.

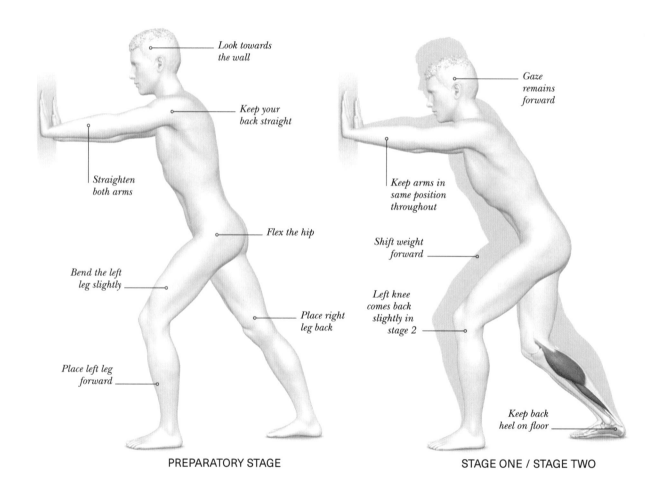

Look towards the wall

Keep your back straight

Straighten both arms

Flex the hip

Bend the left leg slightly

Place right leg back

Place left leg forward

PREPARATORY STAGE

Gaze remains forward

Keep arms in same position throughout

Shift weight forward

Left knee comes back slightly in stage 2

Keep back heel on floor

STAGE ONE / STAGE TWO

PREPARATORY STAGE
Begin in a split stance with your left leg forward, right leg back, and both hands against a wall.

STAGE ONE
Shift your body weight forward over the front leg to achieve a calf stretch in the back leg. Keep the back heel in contact with the floor.

STAGE TWO
Bend the back knee and let your body weight follow. This will shift the stretch to the target muscle. Try to keep the back heel on the floor.

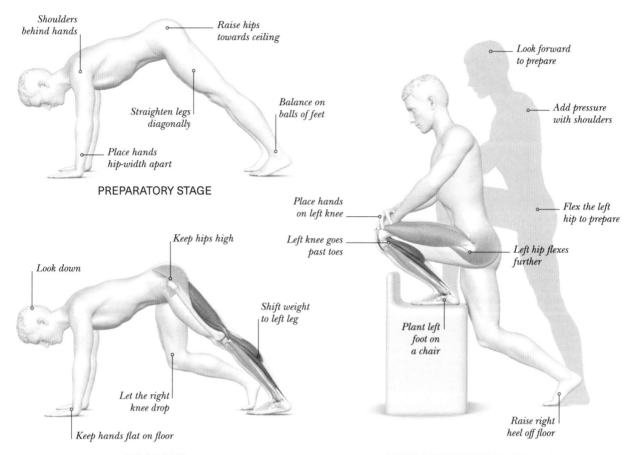

Shoulders behind hands

Raise hips towards ceiling

Straighten legs diagonally

Balance on balls of feet

Place hands hip-width apart

PREPARATORY STAGE

Look forward to prepare

Add pressure with shoulders

Place hands on left knee

Left knee goes past toes

Flex the left hip to prepare

Left hip flexes further

Plant left foot on a chair

Keep hips high

Look down

Shift weight to left leg

Let the right knee drop

Keep hands flat on floor

Raise right heel off floor

STAGE ONE

PREPARATORY STAGE / STAGE ONE

DOWNWARD DOG ALTERNATING KNEE BEND

You can perform this dynamic calf stretch as part of a warmup prior to exercise or sport. It involves assuming a modified "downward dog" position and gently alternating stretches between legs.

PREPARATORY STAGE
Begin on your hands and feet with hips hiked up, knees extended, and heels off the floor, resting on the balls of your feet.

STAGE ONE
Shift the weight to the left leg and let the right knee drop, maintaining the pressure through a straight left leg. Hold for a few seconds.

STAGE TWO
Shift the weight to the right leg, dropping the left knee, and continue to "walk the dog", alternating legs and building a rhythm.

ANKLE DORSIFLEXION ROCK

This exercise is great for exploring ankle dorsiflexion mobility, which is important in daily life and for healthy ankle and knee function. Practise the stretch before exercise to help prepare the ankle joint for motions such as squats or running.

PREPARATORY STAGE
Begin with your left foot on a chair or bench and your right leg on the floor. Rest both hands on the left knee.

STAGE ONE
Slowly bring the knee all the way over the toes to feel a stretch at the end of the movement, while keeping the left heel on the chair.

STAGE TWO
Straighten yourself back up to the preparatory pose with your right heel back on the floor.

KNEELING TOE FLEXOR STRETCH

This exercise is great for gaining some gentle toe extension mobility by stretching the toe flexors. The quadruped position allows for controlled weight through the joint, which can be helpful for stiffer toes.

The powerful flexor hallucis longus muscle crosses the ankle and flexes the great toe. But on the plantar surface of the foot – the thick tissue on the bottom of the foot – there are foot muscles organized in four layers, with the exception of one located on the top of the foot. These muscles are responsible for fine movement of the toes. They also support the arches, and help with posture when walking.

 Caution
Avoid this stretch if you are hypermobile. Pushing end-range stretches can be counterproductive for those with this mobility issue. Be mindful of any foot or ankle pain. Stay within a pain-free range of motion through each stage.

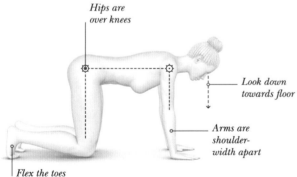

Hips are over knees

Look down towards floor

Arms are shoulder-width apart

Flex the toes

PREPARATORY STAGE
Begin in the four-point kneeling position with the shoulders above the wrists, the hips above the knees, and the head and neck in line. Keep your spine neutral, which refers to the middle, comfortable zone between fully flexed and fully extended. The toes should be tucked under.

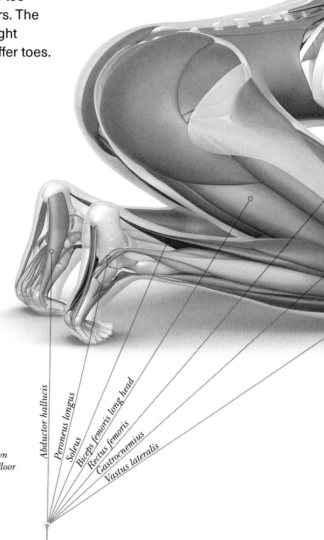

Abductor hallucis
Peroneus longus
Soleus
Biceps femoris long head
Rectus femoris
Gastrocnemius
Vastus lateralis

Lower leg and ankle
The **toe flexors**, including the **flexor hallucis longus** tendon and **intrinsic toe flexors** are lengthened with tension, with the toes in the extended position. The **hamstrings** and **hip flexors** bring the hips towards the feet and flex the knees while controlling stretch intensity.

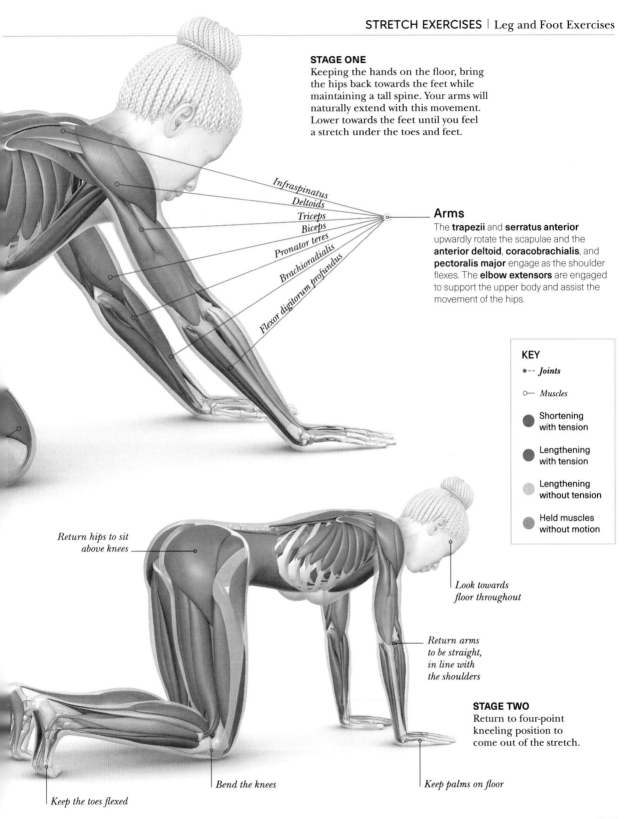

STAGE ONE
Keeping the hands on the floor, bring the hips back towards the feet while maintaining a tall spine. Your arms will naturally extend with this movement. Lower towards the feet until you feel a stretch under the toes and feet.

Infraspinatus
Deltoids
Triceps
Biceps
Pronator teres
Brachioradialis
Flexor digitorum profundus

Arms
The **trapezii** and **serratus anterior** upwardly rotate the scapulae and the **anterior deltoid**, **coracobrachialis**, and **pectoralis major** engage as the shoulder flexes. The **elbow extensors** are engaged to support the upper body and assist the movement of the hips.

KEY

●-- *Joints*

○— *Muscles*

● Shortening with tension

● Lengthening with tension

● Lengthening without tension

● Held muscles without motion

Return hips to sit above knees

Look towards floor throughout

Return arms to be straight, in line with the shoulders

STAGE TWO
Return to four-point kneeling position to come out of the stretch.

Bend the knees

Keep palms on floor

Keep the toes flexed

171

» VARIATIONS

The foot muscles and plantar fascia – tissue that connects the heel bone with the base of your toes – assist us while we stand and walk. These variations improve mobility for daily movement.

TOE WALL STRETCH

This standing variation is an easy way to stretch the toe flexors to gain toe extension mobility. Standing toe flexion is beneficial for activities such as walking and running.

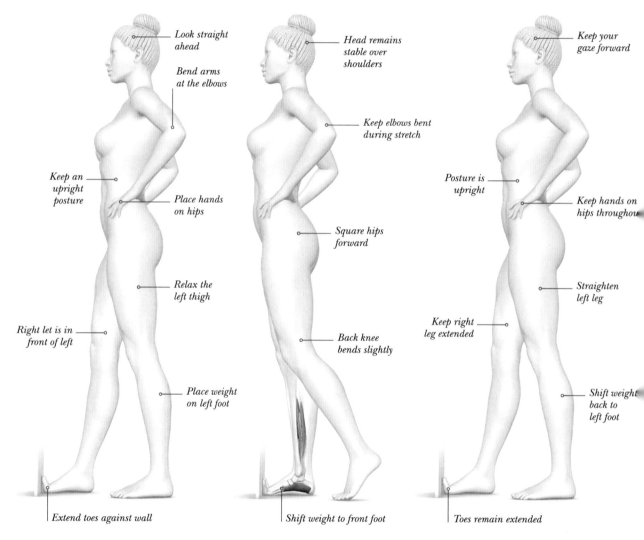

Look straight ahead

Bend arms at the elbows

Keep an upright posture

Place hands on hips

Relax the left thigh

Right let is in front of left

Place weight on left foot

Extend toes against wall

Head remains stable over shoulders

Keep elbows bent during stretch

Square hips forward

Back knee bends slightly

Shift weight to front foot

Keep your gaze forward

Posture is upright

Keep hands on hips throughout

Straighten left leg

Keep right leg extended

Shift weight back to left foot

Toes remain extended

PREPARATORY STAGE
Begin with the toes of your right foot lightly extended against a wall with your weight on the left foot. Place your hands on your hips.

STAGE ONE
Shift your weight forward to the front foot to achieve a greater extension stretch.

STAGE TWO
Shift the weight to the back foot to come out of the stretch.

BENT-KNEE WALL STRETCH

This toe stretch addresses the plantar fascia. Bending the knee achieves greater ankle dorsiflexion, making it a great option to give this area of tissue a good stretch. Incorporate the Bent-knee Wall Stretch into your routine to target foot strength and mobility.

Caution
Avoid this stretch if you are hypermobile. Pushing end-range stretches can be counterproductive for those with this type of mobility. Watch out for any foot or ankle pain, and stay within a pain-free range of motion through each stage.

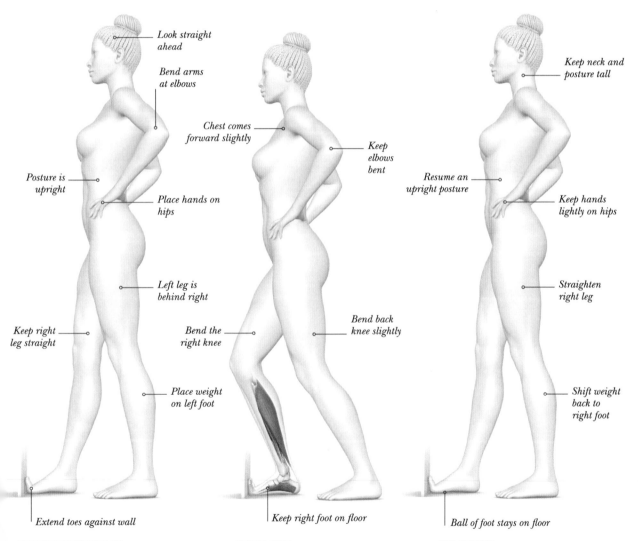

Look straight ahead

Bend arms at elbows

Chest comes forward slightly

Keep elbows bent

Posture is upright

Place hands on hips

Keep neck and posture tall

Resume an upright posture

Keep hands lightly on hips

Left leg is behind right

Keep right leg straight

Bend the right knee

Bend back knee slightly

Straighten right leg

Place weight on left foot

Shift weight back to right foot

Extend toes against wall

Keep right foot on floor

Ball of foot stays on floor

PREPARATORY STAGE
Begin with the toes of your right foot lightly extended against the wall with your weight on the left foot.

STAGE ONE
Bend the right knee and drive it forward while keeping the right heel flat on the floor.

STAGE TWO
Shift the weight to the back foot to come out of the stretch.

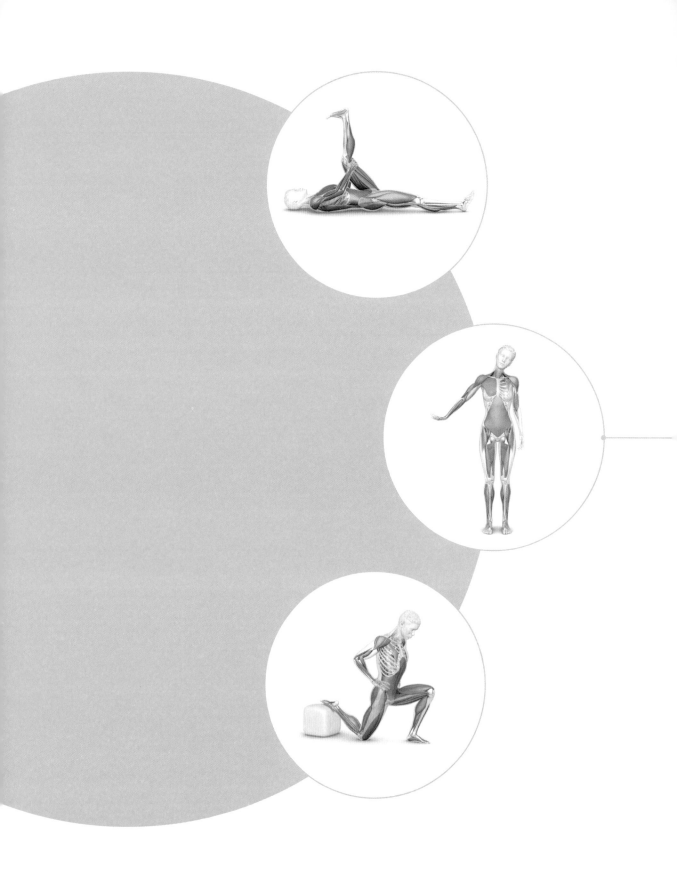

NERVE MOBILITY EXERCISES

How the nervous system communicates with itself and relates to the musculoskeletal system can affect movement and range of motion, as well as causing symptoms like tightness. Use these stretches to target nerve mobility in the main nerves in the upper and lower extremities, such as the median nerve, running down the anterior arm, and the sciatic nerve, running down each leg from the lower back.

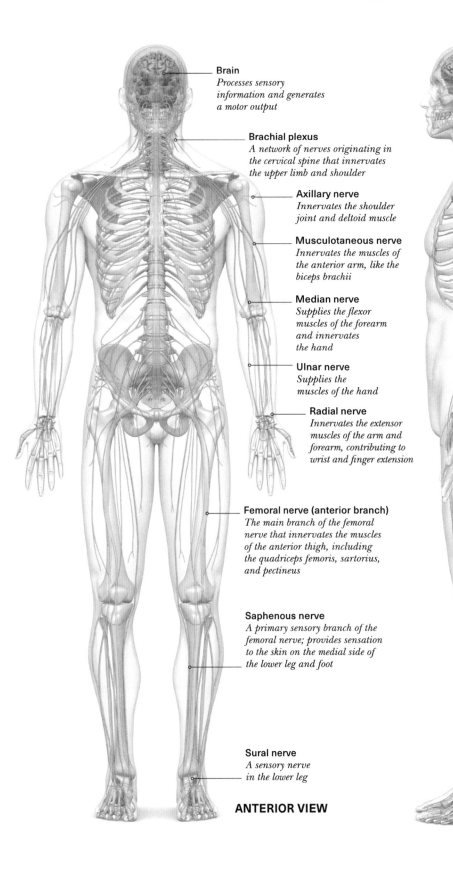

Brain
*Processes sensory
information and generates
a motor output*

Brachial plexus
*A network of nerves originating in
the cervical spine that innervates
the upper limb and shoulder*

Axillary nerve
*Innervates the shoulder
joint and deltoid muscle*

Musculotaneous nerve
*Innervates the muscles of
the anterior arm, like the
biceps brachii*

Median nerve
*Supplies the flexor
muscles of the forearm
and innervates
the hand*

Ulnar nerve
*Supplies the
muscles of the hand*

Radial nerve
*Innervates the extensor
muscles of the arm and
forearm, contributing to
wrist and finger extension*

Femoral nerve (anterior branch)
*The main branch of the femoral
nerve that innervates the muscles
of the anterior thigh, including
the quadriceps femoris, sartorius,
and pectineus*

Saphenous nerve
*A primary sensory branch of the
femoral nerve; provides sensation
to the skin on the medial side of
the lower leg and foot*

Sural nerve
*A sensory nerve
in the lower leg*

ANTERIOR VIEW

Brain
*Central command
centre for the
nervous system*

**Brachial plexus
nerve roots**
*The spinal nerves
that make up the
brachial plexus
(C5–T1)*

Femoral nerve
*Supplies sensation to
the front of the thigh
and inner leg*

Sciatic nerve
*The largest nerve in the
body; originates in the
lower back and travels
through the back of the
thigh, supplying the
muscles and skin of the
leg and foot*

Tibial nerve
*A branch of the sciatic
nerve; runs down the
posterior leg and
innervates the posterior
lower leg and foot*

LATERAL VIEW

NERVE MOBILITY OVERVIEW

The nervous system coordinates and controls the body's functions, allowing for communication and response to internal and external stimuli. The main nerves in the arms include the median nerve, ulnar nerve, and radial nerve. In the legs, major nerves include the sciatic nerve, femoral nerve, and tibial nerve.

The median, ulnar, and radial nerves in the arms are responsible for both sensory and motor functions. Sensory information, including touch, temperature, and proprioception, is carried from the skin, joints, and muscles back to the central nervous system via these nerves. Motor signals are transmitted from the central nervous system to the muscles, allowing for voluntary movement and control of the arms. Similarly, in the legs, nerves including the sciatic, femoral, and tibial nerves, and other branches, facilitate sensory input and motor control. These nerves play essential roles in sensation, coordination, and movement of the limbs, contributing to overall body function and interaction with the environment.

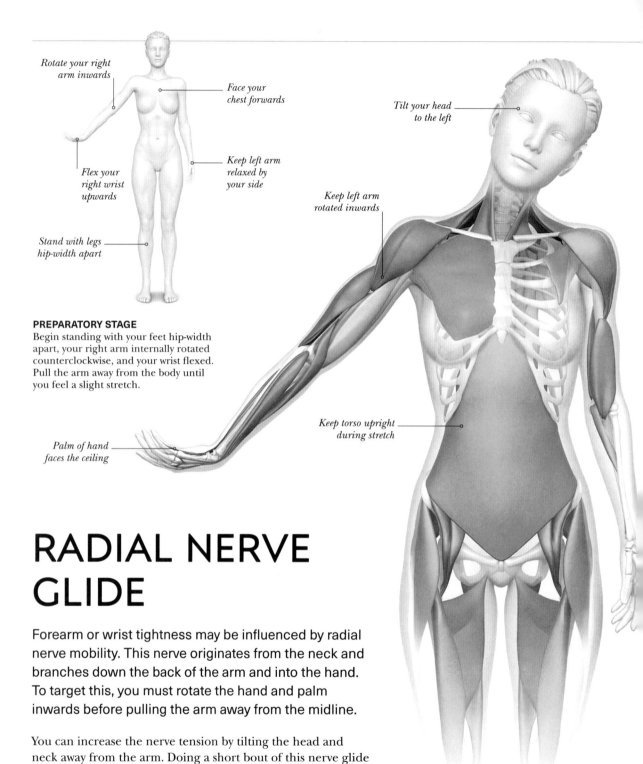

Rotate your right
arm inwards

Face your
chest forwards

Tilt your head
to the left

Flex your
right wrist
upwards

Keep left arm
relaxed by
your side

Keep left arm
rotated inwards

Stand with legs
hip-width apart

PREPARATORY STAGE
Begin standing with your feet hip-width
apart, your right arm internally rotated
counterclockwise, and your wrist flexed.
Pull the arm away from the body until
you feel a slight stretch.

Keep torso upright
during stretch

Palm of hand
faces the ceiling

RADIAL NERVE GLIDE

Forearm or wrist tightness may be influenced by radial
nerve mobility. This nerve originates from the neck and
branches down the back of the arm and into the hand.
To target this, you must rotate the hand and palm
inwards before pulling the arm away from the midline.

You can increase the nerve tension by tilting the head and
neck away from the arm. Doing a short bout of this nerve glide
may help reduce posterior arm tightness due to nerve-related
stiffness, and can help reduce forearm tension. Perform with
caution if you have neck pain or a history of nerve pain.

STAGE ONE
Tilt the neck to the left, away from
the arm, to increase the stretch.

Neck and arm

The **right scalenes** and **sternocleidomastoid** are lengthened. The **subscapularis** and **pectorals** internally rotate the shoulder, while the **triceps** maintain elbow extension. The **pronator teres** and **pronator quadratus** engage to pronate the forearm.

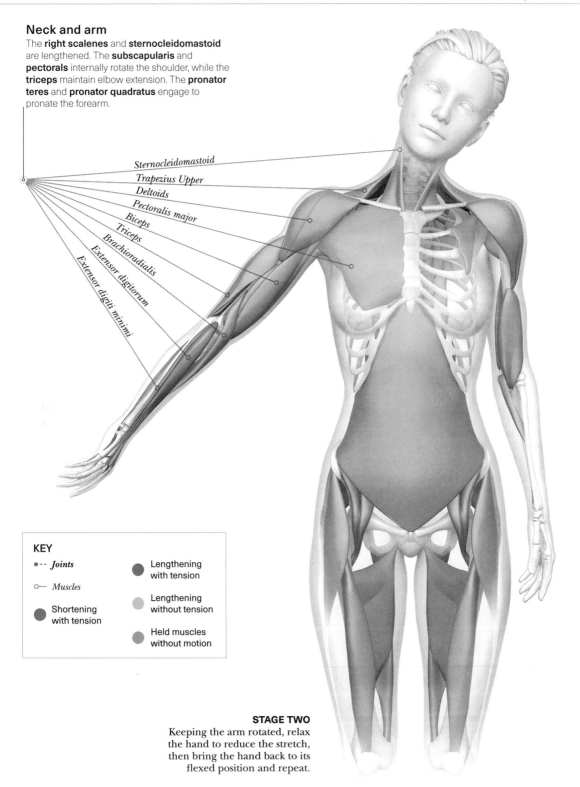

Sternocleidomastoid
Trapezius Upper
Deltoids
Pectoralis major
Biceps
Triceps
Brachioradialis
Extensor digitorum
Extensor digiti minimi

KEY

•-- *Joints*

○— *Muscles*

● Shortening with tension

● Lengthening with tension

● Lengthening without tension

● Held muscles without motion

STAGE TWO
Keeping the arm rotated, relax the hand to reduce the stretch, then bring the hand back to its flexed position and repeat.

» VARIATIONS

There are many nerves that exist throughout the arm, wrist, and hand area. The main nerves in these areas have unique pathways that power specific muscles.

MEDIAN NERVE GLIDE

Forearm or wrist tightness may be influenced by median nerve mobility. This nerve originates from the neck and branches down the anterior arm. To target this, you must rotate the hand and palm outwards, extend the wrist, and pull the arm away from the midline. Increase the nerve tension by tilting the head and neck away from the arm. This stretch may help reduce tension in the wrist and forearm.

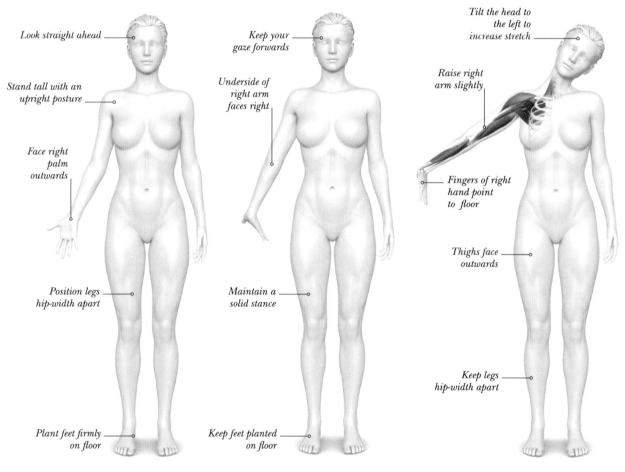

Look straight ahead

Stand tall with an upright posture

Face right palm outwards

Position legs hip-width apart

Plant feet firmly on floor

Keep your gaze forwards

Underside of right arm faces right

Maintain a solid stance

Keep feet planted on floor

Tilt the head to the left to increase stretch

Raise right arm slightly

Fingers of right hand point to floor

Thighs face outwards

Keep legs hip-width apart

PREPARATORY STAGE
Begin standing tall with the right arm and palm facing forward.

STAGE ONE
Rotate the arm away from the midline so that the underside of the arm faces right, and pull the wrist back.

STAGE TWO
Raise the right arm slightly and tilt the head to the left to increase the stretch, then bring the wrist back to the neutral preparatory position.

ULNAR NERVE GLIDE

Forearm or wrist tightness may be influenced by ulnar nerve mobility. This nerve originates from the neck and branches down the medial elbow and last two fingers. It's often referred to as the "funny bone". To target this, you must pronate the hand and palm downwards with a flexed shoulder and bent elbow. You can increase the nerve tension by tilting the head and neck away from the arm. Doing a short bout of this nerve glide may help posterior arm tightness due to nerve-related stiffness, and address any forearm tension.

! Caution

Avoid this stretch if you have acute neck pain. Be mindful of excessive discomfort or pain in the forearm, shoulder, or neck. This should feel like a comfortable movement through the back of the arm. Stay within a pain-free range of motion through each stage. At most it should feel like a slight deep pull in stage 1, with relief at stage 2. Stop if you have any excessive numbness, tingling, or pain.

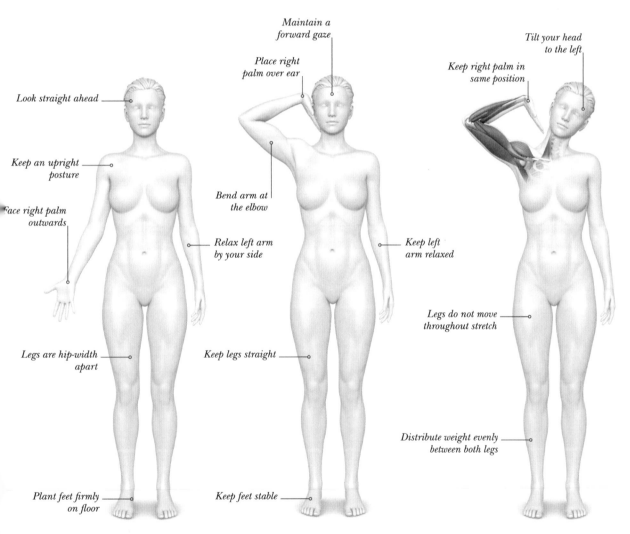

Look straight ahead

Keep an upright posture

Face right palm outwards

Legs are hip-width apart

Plant feet firmly on floor

Maintain a forward gaze

Place right palm over ear

Bend arm at the elbow

Relax left arm by your side

Keep legs straight

Keep feet stable

Tilt your head to the left

Keep right palm in same position

Keep left arm relaxed

Legs do not move throughout stretch

Distribute weight evenly between both legs

PREPARATORY STAGE
Begin standing with the right arm and palm facing forward.

STAGE ONE
Turn the palm downwards and bring the right arm up by the ear with the fingers down, as if to cover your ear. Only move into the range as far as you can tolerate.

STAGE TWO
Tilt the head away from your hand to the left to increase the stretch.

SCIATIC NERVE GLIDE

Limited sciatic nerve mobility may contribute to discomfort in the back of the thigh or leg. One way to mobilize this nerve is to flex the hip, extend the knee, and move the ankle up and down.

You can increase the nerve tension by flexing the head and neck. Doing a short bout of this nerve glide may help reduce posterior hip and thigh pain due to nerve-related perceived tightness, may help reduce hamstring or calf tension, and can address hip and knee range of motion. The nerve glide can be done with sustained knee flexion ankle movement, or by coordinating active knee extension. Note that the straighter the knee is with ankle dorsiflexion, the greater the nerve is tensioned.

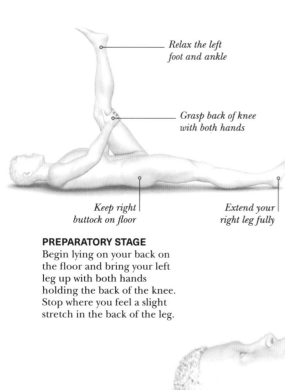

Relax the left foot and ankle

Grasp back of knee with both hands

Keep right buttock on floor

Extend your right leg fully

PREPARATORY STAGE
Begin lying on your back on the floor and bring your left leg up with both hands holding the back of the knee. Stop where you feel a slight stretch in the back of the leg.

STAGE ONE
Flex the left foot and toes towards the head to increase the stretch in the nerve.

Arms
The **biceps brachii, brachialis,** and **brachioradialis** flex the elbow. The **wrist** and **finger flexors** are engaged to hold the leg. The **diaphragm** leads to relaxed breathing.

Extensor digitorum
Brachioradialis
Flexor digitorum profundus
Triceps
Brachialis
Biceps
Deltoids

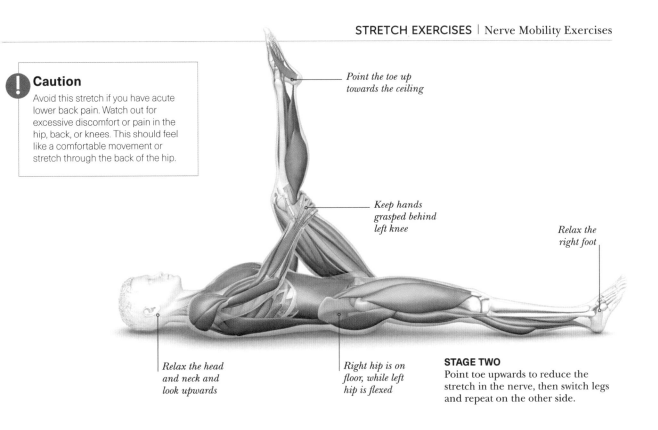

Caution

Avoid this stretch if you have acute lower back pain. Watch out for excessive discomfort or pain in the hip, back, or knees. This should feel like a comfortable movement or stretch through the back of the hip.

Point the toe up towards the ceiling

Keep hands grasped behind left knee

Relax the right foot

Relax the head and neck and look upwards

Right hip is on floor, while left hip is flexed

STAGE TWO
Point toe upwards to reduce the stretch in the nerve, then switch legs and repeat on the other side.

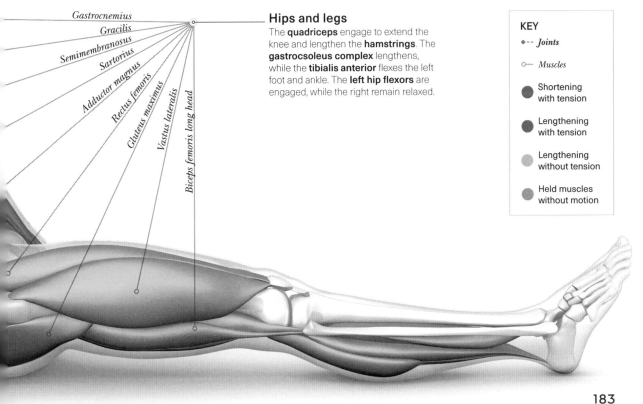

Gastrocnemius
Gracilis
Semimembranosus
Sartorius
Adductor magnus
Rectus femoris
Gluteus maximus
Vastus lateralis
Biceps femoris long head

Hips and legs

The **quadriceps** engage to extend the knee and lengthen the **hamstrings**. The **gastrocsoleus complex** lengthens, while the **tibialis anterior** flexes the left foot and ankle. The **left hip flexors** are engaged, while the right remain relaxed.

KEY

● -- *Joints*

○— *Muscles*

● Shortening with tension

● Lengthening with tension

● Lengthening without tension

● Held muscles without motion

» VARIATIONS

The sciatic nerve divides into the tibial and fibular nerves. A branch from each of these combine to form the sural nerve, which provides sensory function to the lower leg, foot, and ankle.

TIBIAL NERVE GLIDE

Using more specific nerve glides may help with complaints in various regions of the leg. The tibial nerve is a branch of the sciatic nerve that runs along the inside of the ankle. In order to mobilize this nerve, the hip has to be flexed, with the knee extended and the ankle moving up and away from the body (dorsiflexion and eversion). You can increase the nerve tension by flexing your neck up towards the foot.

! Caution

Avoid this stretch if you have acute lower back pain. Be mindful of excessive discomfort or pain in the hip, back, or knees.

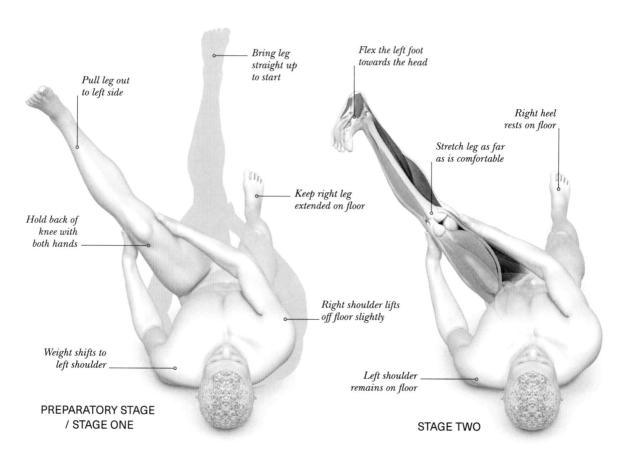

Pull leg out to left side

Bring leg straight up to start

Flex the left foot towards the head

Right heel rests on floor

Stretch leg as far as is comfortable

Keep right leg extended on floor

Hold back of knee with both hands

Right shoulder lifts off floor slightly

Weight shifts to left shoulder

Left shoulder remains on floor

PREPARATORY STAGE / STAGE ONE

STAGE TWO

PREPARATORY STAGE
Begin lying on the floor. Bring your left leg up and hold the back of the knee with both hands. Extend the knee to feel a stretch behind the thigh.

STAGE ONE
Pull the leg out to the left and away from the midline by abducting the hip, keeping your pelvis and back flat on the floor.

STAGE TWO
Flex the left foot up towards the head and away from the midline to complete the stretch.

FIBULAR NERVE GLIDE

The fibular nerve is a branch of the sciatic nerve that runs along the outside of the lower leg and ankle, and supplies muscles in the lateral compartment of the lower leg. To mobilize this nerve, you flex the hip, with the knee extended and the ankle moving up and towards the body. To increase the tension of the nerve, flex the neck up towards the foot.

PREPARATORY STAGE
Begin lying on your back and bring your left leg up, with two hands holding the back of the knee. Extend the knee until you feel a stretch behind the thigh.

STAGE ONE
Pull the leg to the right towards the midline by adducting the hip. Keep the pelvis and back flat on the floor.

STAGE TWO
Flex the foot up towards the head and towards the midline to complete the stretch.

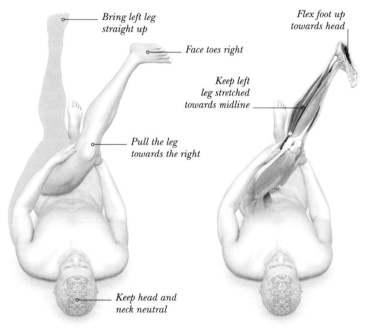

Bring left leg straight up

Face toes right

Pull the leg towards the right

Keep head and neck neutral

Flex foot up towards head

Keep left leg stretched towards midline

PREPARATORY STAGE / STAGE ONE

STAGE TWO

SURAL NERVE GLIDE

The sural nerve is a branch of the sciatic nerve that runs along the back and outside of the lower leg and ankle. To mobilize this nerve while lying on your back, you flex the hip with the knee extended and ankle moving down and towards the body (plantarflexion and inversion). If you find the stretch easy, increase the nerve tension by flexing the neck up towards the foot.

PREPARATORY STAGE
Begin lying on your back. Bring your left leg up and hold the back of the knee with both hands. Extend the knee to the where you feel a stretch behind the thigh.

STAGE ONE
Pull the left leg to the right and towards the midline by adducting the hip. Keep the pelvis and back flat on the floor.

STAGE TWO
Point the foot down and inwards to complete the movement.

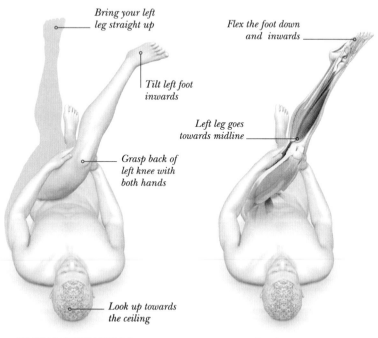

Bring your left leg straight up

Tilt left foot inwards

Grasp back of left knee with both hands

Look up towards the ceiling

Flex the foot down and inwards

Left leg goes towards midline

PREPARATORY STAGE / STAGE ONE

STAGE TWO

185

FEMORAL NERVE GLIDE

The femoral nerve supplies nerves to the thigh and hip muscles that flex the hip and extend the knee. To tense the femoral nerve, the hip must be extended and the knee flexed, as in this stretch.

Symptoms related to the femoral nerve may typically present near the anterior thigh or leg. Performing a short bout of this nerve glide may help reduce anterior hip tightness due to neural tension, may help improve hip extension range of motion, and reduce any discomfort at the anterior thigh. You can increase the nerve tension by looking down or up with the head and neck.

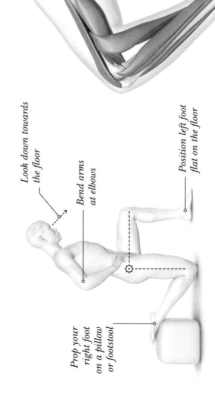

Look down towards the floor

Bend arms at elbows

Position left foot flat on the floor

Prop your right foot on a pillow or footstool

PREPARATORY STAGE
Begin in a half-kneeling position with your left leg in front, and your rear ankle propped on a pillow or footstool. Keep your spine neutral and gaze down. You should feel a stretch in the hip flexor and in the front of the thigh.

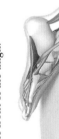

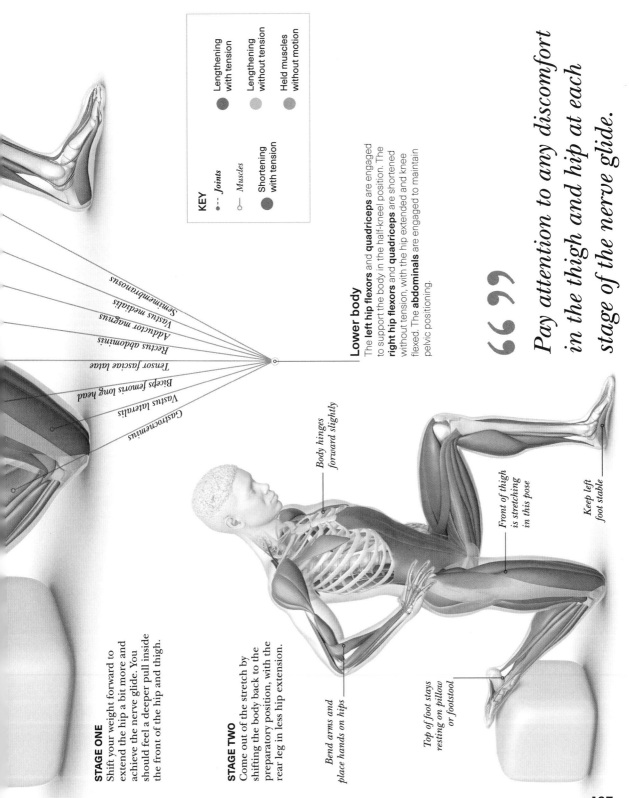

STAGE ONE

Shift your weight forward to extend the hip a bit more and achieve the nerve glide. You should feel a deeper pull inside the front of the hip and thigh.

STAGE TWO

Come out of the stretch by shifting the body back to the preparatory position, with the rear leg in less hip extension.

KEY

- - - *Joints*

○— *Muscles*

● Shortening with tension

● Lengthening with tension

● Lengthening without tension

● Held muscles without motion

Gastrocnemius

Vastus lateralis

Biceps femoris long head

Tensor fasciae latae

Rectus abdominis

Adductor magnus

Vastus medialis

Semimembranosus

Lower body

The **left hip flexors** and **quadriceps** are engaged to support the body in the half-kneel position. The **right hip flexors** and **quadriceps** are shortened without tension, with the hip extended and knee flexed. The **abdominals** are engaged to maintain pelvic positioning.

❝❞

Pay attention to any discomfort in the thigh and hip at each stage of the nerve glide.

Body hinges forward slightly

Front of thigh is stretching in this pose

Keep left foot stable

Bend arms and place hands on hips

Top of foot stays resting on pillow or footstool

STRETCH
ROUTINES

Central to achieving physical activity goals is building a programme tailored to your choice of movement. You may wish to enhance your sports training – strength training or a myriad of other sports – to achieve a more active lifestyle. You may want to target a part of the body, such as the spine, or hips and knees, or you may want to stretch your whole body in a full body routine. Organized into easy-to follow lists, and arranged into beginner and advanced sections, these suggested routines can assist in taking that extra step towards purposeful movement exploration.

INTRODUCTION TO THE ROUTINES

There is a variety of stretches in this book suitable for many levels. As you explore your mobility and work to improve flexibility and general physical wellbeing, remember to modify as needed and listen to your body.

Stretching research continues to evolve and the optimal stretch dosage will vary per person, activity, and experience level. Studies have investigated the effects of different stretch dosages on various outcomes, such as range of motion and muscle soreness. The following sections provide suggested guidelines for stretching based on goals and experience.

BEGINNER

Beginners can start to train flexibility by incorporating stretches once per day, three to five days a week. Start with a light warmup of low-intensity activity to warm up the muscles. You can hold static stretches for up to 30 seconds and target major muscle groups.

Stretches may be pushed to slight discomfort, but should not elicit any lingering pain. Paying attention to sensations and tolerance will help improve your body awareness. As flexibility increases, sensations may change, and new ranges will need to be targeted for further change.

As you feel more comfortable, gradually increase the intensity or duration to progress. Practise relaxed and controlled breathing during stretches, and seek guidance from a qualified professional for personalized instruction and to address specific concerns. Remember, consistency is important for adaptation.

ADVANCED

Those with more movement or sports experience may choose to partake in more advanced stretches. These stretches can include multiple muscle groups at once and be multiplanar in nature (p.14). Assess current flexibility levels and identify areas of focus that require further improvement or maintenance. Start with an active warmup that includes dynamic movements to target specific muscle groups. Advanced stretches will likely be dynamic and mimic the subsequent activity. Stretch techniques like PNF stretching or eccentric movements can be used (p.42), which are more intense and may require assistance or equipment. The duration and intensity of stretches for the advanced mover can be longer to challenge the muscles more, especially if done for sports that require a lot of flexibility, like martial arts or dance. Since greater-intensity stretches can yield greater ranges of motion, it should be noted

Beginner

Static stretches:
1–2 sets of 15–30 seconds

Dynamic stretches:
1–2 sets of 10–15 reps at 1–2 second holds

Target major muscle groups and opt for simple one- to two-joint muscles to stretch, like the hamstrings or calves. Get accustomed to the sensations and positions to learn body awareness. Pay attention to what you feel during and after the stretch, as well as the following day. Perform at least 3 times per week, ideally as part of a greater exercise routine.

Advanced

Static stretches:
1–3 sets of 15–60 seconds

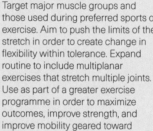

Dynamic stretches:
1–2 sets of 10–20 reps at 1–2 second holds

Target major muscle groups and those used during preferred sports or exercise. Aim to push the limits of the stretch in order to create change in flexibility within tolerance. Expand routine to include multiplanar exercises that stretch multiple joints. Use as part of a greater exercise programme in order to maximize outcomes, improve strength, and improve mobility geared toward movement and exercise goals.

Static stretches
These involve holding a muscle or joint in one fixed position, e.g.:
Child's Pose p.78
Cobra p.80
Seated Butterfly Stretch p.146

Dynamic stretches
These involve moving a muscle or joint through its full range of motion, e.g.:
Cat Cow p.74
Thread the Needle p.94
World's Greatest Stretch p.140

that strength training in these ranges is also beneficial to best reduce injury. Additionally, proper recovery and exercise programming is of key importance. Advanced participants should continue to listen to their bodies and avoid pushing into excessive discomfort.

STATIC VS DYNAMIC

Static and dynamic stretches are two types of stretching that vary mainly by the duration of holds. Both can improve range of motion. Static stretches involve holding a stretch for a prolonged period, typically 15 to 60 seconds. The muscle is gradually lengthened and held at its maximum point of tension. It is commonly performed after physical activity or as part of a flexibility or mobility training programme. Static stretches may be better suited for the beginner as they are often simpler movements. Dynamic stretches involve controlled, repetitive movements that take a joint or muscle through its full range of motion, holding for 1 to 2 seconds, or less than 15 seconds. They require coordination and can improve dynamic joint stability, neuromuscular control, and muscular performance. If done as part of a dynamic warmup, stretches can be executed at normal or faster speeds within the available range of motion. They can also be done at normal speeds towards the end of the range to train flexibility. The dynamic warmups that follow are created with dynamic stretches, although the same stretches may be listed as static elsewhere (i.e. mobility). Ultimately, the stretch type will depend on goals.

A mixture of static and dynamic stretches is given. Do static stretches to enhance flexibility, and dynamic stretches to prepare the body for physical activity.

SIMPLE TIPS TO REMEMBER

Consider these points when embarking on your flexibility journey.

- **Warm up** before stretching to increase blood flow to muscles.
- **Choose stretch types** relevant to movement goals.
- **Start gently**, gradually increasing intensity and duration of stretches.
- **Try** both active and passive stretches. Active stretches focus on using one muscle group to stretch another; passive stretches use an external force like another part of the body or a partner.
- **Strengthen** the appropriate muscles by building in strength training sessions alongside stretching, targeted at muscles relevant to your goals.
- **Be consistent:** perform 3 to 5 days per week.
- **Modify** if you experience prolonged discomfort, and seek guidance from a qualified professional if needed.

66 99

Both static and dynamic stretching can improve range of motion. Which you choose to utilize will depend on your goals and activity.

NECK AND SHOULDER ROUTINES

The muscles of the neck and shoulder region are typically areas where people seek help – for pain relief or to maintain of regular range of motion. However, the thoracic spine is an area that can also contribute to mobility here as well.

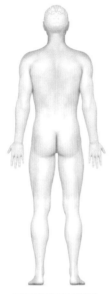

POSTERIOR VIEW

The main muscles that control the neck include the periscapular, sternocleidomastoid, and suboccipital muscles, as well as the scalenes, deep neck stabilizers, and neck extensors. Because the neck and shoulder muscles are related, it's not uncommon for people to experience symptoms like perceived tightness in a neighbouring area with pain, overuse, or injury. Nerve irritations at the level of the neck or neck-specific injuries can contribute to symptoms in the arm or scapular region. In these cases, stretching may not be appropriate: be sure to get evaluated. In the cases of basic range of motion, stretching exercises can target the neck, shoulders, thoracic spine, and contributing muscles. Remember to pair with strength exercises for the relevant muscles.

Beginner

Static stretches:
Hold 15–30 seconds
Dynamic stretches (D):
Do 10–15 reps at 1–2 second holds

---
1. Levator Stretch p.68

---
2. Manual Suboccipital Stretch p.69

---
3. Sternocleidomastoid Stretch p.70

---
4. Scalene Stretch p.72

---
5. Doorway Pec Stretch p.102

---
6. Seated Cat Cow (D) p.75

---
7. Cross Body Glute Stretch p.130

Advanced

Dynamic stretches:
Do 10–15 reps at 1–2 second holds

---
1. Thread the Needle: Hand Behind Head p.96

---
2. Standing Half Moon p.92

---
3. Puppy Pose p.86

---
4. Floor Angel p.106

---
5. Standing Thoracic Extension Wall Stretch p.84

---
6. Thread the Needle p.94

---
7. Cat Cow p.74

SPINE ROUTINES

Stretches focussing on the spine will include flexion, extension, side bend, and rotational motions. These motions may be a priority for maintenance or be targeted in relation to a sport or activity.

The spine supports the body and protects the spinal cord. Regular stretching exercises targeted to this particular region can help to maintain the range of motion, which is imperative for many sports. However, be sure to always stay within a comfortable range.

EXERCISE SELECTION
Choosing the right stretch will depend on your comfort level and abilities. The neck typically has the most range of motion available, followed by the upper back and, lastly, the lower back. Incorporating a variety of spine stretches into your stretching routine can help maintain spinal health, alleviate back pain, and promote overall wellbeing. It's important to perform spine stretches with guided technique and to honour your body's limitations. Age-related changes in the spine like spinal stenosis or osteoporosis can limit range of motion, so be sure to modify or stay within a comfortable range – ask your healthcare provider for the best plan to cater to your needs.

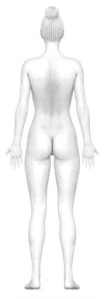

POSTERIOR VIEW

Beginner

Static stretches:
Hold 15–30 seconds

Dynamic stretches (D):
Do 10–15 reps at 1–2 second holds

1. Cat Cow (D) p.74

2. Thread the Needle (D) p.94

3. Child's Pose p.78

4. Cobra p.80

5. Standing Thoracic Extension Wall Stretch (D) p.84

6. Half Moon on Floor (D) p.93

7. Standing Thoracic Extension: Arms on Chair (D) p.86

Advanced

Static stretches:
Hold 15–30 seconds

Dynamic stretches (D):
Do 10–15 reps at 1–2 second holds

1. Child's Pose: Lateral p.79

2. Standing Thoracic Extension: Arms on Chair (D) p.86

3. Half-Kneel Thoracic Rotation (D) p.88

4. Thread the Needle (D) p.94

5. Thread the Needle: Hand Behind Head (D) p.96

6. Half Moon on Floor (D) p.93

7. Bretzel p.91

" "

Different regions of the spine are capable of more or less motion, but each region is able to flex, extend, and rotate.

HIP AND KNEE ROUTINES

Mobility at the hips and knees, and how they function with the foot and ankle, play an important role in how we walk, run, and move. While it's imprtant to keep the joint mobile, the muscles around it are targeted for strength and flexibility.

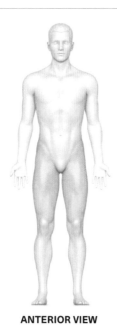

ANTERIOR VIEW

The glutes, hip abductors, hip flexors, quadriceps, hamstrings, and hip rotators are the main muscles that influence the hip and knee. The core muscles can influence the pelvis, and the gastrocnemius also influences the knee because it crosses the joint.

These muscles are critical for locomotion throughout the lifespan and are especially important in functional movement, such as squats, lunging, and jumping. Hip flexor and hamstring flexibility can be helpful for walking and running and contribute to improved sports performance. While needs may vary depending on factors such as age, activity level, and specific sport or activity requirements, good flexibility in these joints allows for proper form, effective movement patterns, and reduced stress on the joints and surrounding tissues.

Beginner

Static stretches:
Hold 15–30 seconds

1. Figure 4 Stretch p.128

2. Cross Body Glute Stretch p.130

3. Standing Hip Flexor Stretch p.136

4. Pancake Stretch p.142

5. Seated Butterfly Stretch p.146

6. Standing Quad Stretch p.156

7. Static Hamstring Stretch p.160

Advanced

Static stretches:
Hold 15–30 seconds

Dynamic stretches (D):
Do 10–15 reps at 1–2 second holds

1. Half-Kneel Hip Flexor Rock (D) p.122

2. Hamstring Rockback (D) p.121

3. Half-Kneel Couch Stretch p.159

4. Figure 4 Hip Internal Rotation Stretch (D) p.132

5. Pigeon Stretch p.138

6. Adductor Rockback (D) p.120

7. Garland Squat (D) p.126

FOOT AND ANKLE ROUTINES

There are many joints in the foot and ankle and numerous muscles that influence them. The muscles of the foot, including the intrinsic and extrinsic muscles, and the ankle, play a crucial role in providing stability, support, and movement to the lower extremities.

The intrinsic foot muscles are located within the foot and are responsible for maintaining the arch, motor control, and providing stability. The extrinsic foot muscles originate on the outside of the foot and lower leg and extend into the ankle. These muscles are responsible for larger movements and provide power and control to actions such as ankle dorsiflexion, plantarflexion, inversion, and eversion (see glossary on p.208 for explanations of these terms).

Overuse, injury, and immobilization can contribute to stiffness in these joints. Calf tightness is correlated to plantar fasciopathy (inflammation on the bottom of your foot, around the heel and arch). Limited big toe extension can influence stability and ankle movement (see p.58).

We may not always consider that feet and ankles need to be exercised, in addition to the rest of the body, but it is crucial to keep these areas strong and flexible, as they bear the weight of the whole body.

Exercises focussed on strengthening and stretching these muscles, when appropriate, can be beneficial for improving foot and ankle function, balance, and overall lower limb performance.

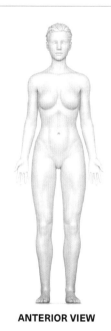

ANTERIOR VIEW

Beginner

Static stretches:
Hold 15–30 seconds

Dynamic stretches (D):
Do 10–15 reps at 1–2 second holds

1. Gastrocnemius Wall Stretch (D) p.166

2. Bent-Knee Calf Stretch p.168

3. Toe Wall Stretch p.172

4. Ankle Dorsiflexion Rock (D) p.169

Advanced

Static stretches:
Hold 15–30 seconds

Dynamic stretches (D):
Do 10–15 reps at 1–2 second holds

1. Gastrocnemius Step Stretch (D) p.164

2. Downward Dog Alternating Knee Bend (D) p.169

3. Kneeling Toe Flexor Stretch p.170

4. Bent-Knee Wall Stretch p.173

FULL BODY ROUTINES

Simple, full body stretch routines can feel great and are a nice way to include low-intensity movement as a standalone, as part of a greater routine, or to maintain general mobility. Their short nature makes them easy to stay consistent with training.

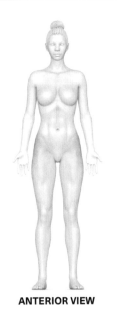

ANTERIOR VIEW

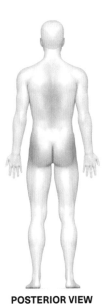

POSTERIOR VIEW

A full body routine can be catered to individual needs, but can generally be built around areas that affect daily movement the most, like the hips, or those that don't stretch often, like the thoracic spine.

CONSISTENCY MATTERS

Our joints will maintain their range of motion so long as we continue to move and exercise regularly. This can be done with stretching and strengthening through full ranges of motion. Full body routines can offer structure and maintenance to keep the body mobile in ways that affect us the most.

The routines offered here are sample programmes, but you can experiment and explore your options by including different stretches for relevant joints. A good rule of thumb in creating your own full body routine is to include one to two stretches per major muscle group or region. This could be hips, shoulders, arms, and hands, legs and feet, or any of the other categories that are outlined in the main part of this book.

Beginner

Static stretches:
Hold 15–30 seconds

Dynamic stretches (D):
Do 10–15 reps at 1–2 second holds

1. Sciatic Nerve Glide (D) p.182

2. Happy Baby Pose p.144

3. Standing Hip Flexor Stretch p.136

4. Standing Thoracic Rotation (D) p.90

5. Cobra p.80

6. Child's Pose (with lateral variation) p.78

7. Cat Cow (D) p.74

Advanced

Static stretches:
Hold 15–30 seconds

Dynamic stretches (D):
Do 10–15 reps at 1–2 second holds

1. Downward Dog Alternating Knee Bend (D) p.169

2. Hamstring Rockback (D) p.121

3. Thread the Needle in Adductor Stretch (D) p.96

4. Quadratus Lumborum Stretch p.76

5. Standing Thoracic Extension Wall Stretch (D) p.84

6. World's Greatest Stretch (D) p.140

7. Garland Squat (D) p.126

PELVIC FLOOR RELAXATION

A hyperactive pelvic floor can be present with issues like hip, back, and pelvic pain; urinary symptoms or bowel dysfunction; and sexual dysfunction. The pelvic floor muscles line the bottom of the pelvis and coordinate with the breathing muscles, like the diaphragm, for optimal breathing mechanics and core stability during various activities, including exercise, lifting heavy objects, or everyday movements. You can train these muscles to strengthen or relax, depending on individual needs.

Exhale and relax the pelvic floor during these stretches, especially those that include hip and pelvic positioning, to facilitate lengthening of the pelvic muscles. Consult a pelvic floor physical therapist for individual needs.

Basic Relaxation

Static stretches:
Hold 15–30 seconds

Dynamic streches (D):
Do 10–15 reps at 1–2 second holds

1. Cat Cow (D) p.74

2. Child's Pose p.78

3. Adductor Rockback (D) p.120

4. Frog Rockback (D) p.121

5. Puppy Pose p.86

6. Figure 4 Stretch p.128

7. Happy Baby Pose p.144

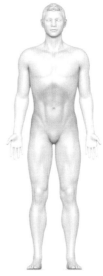

ANTERIOR VIEW

NERVE GLIDES

Nerves course through the muscles and tissues of the body and adapt to loads as we move (see p.31). Neural symptoms like pulling, aching, tingling, or numbness along a limb's nerve can be exacerbated by movement after a period of inactivity, such as injury, or due to irritation along the nerve path or nerve root.

Nerve mobilizations, often called "nerve glides" or "nerve flossing" can help promote healthy neural movement and reduce symptoms. Pair with relevant dynamic movement to similar joints. Consult a professional for individual needs.

Upper body

Dynamic stretches:
Do 10–20 reps at
1-2 second holds

1. Radial Nerve Glide p.178

2. Median Nerve Glide p.180

3. Ulnar Nerve Glide p.181

4. Doorway Pec Stretch p.102

5. Standing Half Moon p.92

Lower body

Dynamic stretches:
Do 10–20 reps at
1–2 second holds

1. Sciatic Nerve Glide p.182

2. Tibial Nerve Glide p.184

3. Fibular Nerve Glide p.185

4. Sural Nerve Glide p.185

5. Femoral Nerve Glide p.186

197

ROUTINES FOR DESKBOUND WORKERS

More and more people now work from home and may spend whole days sitting at a desk, with little incentive to get up and move around occasionally.

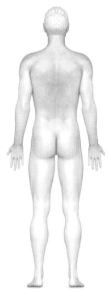

POSTERIOR VIEW

Some of the most common complaints associated with lack of physical activity and prolonged sitting at a desk include neck pain, shoulder pain, and back pain. Light physical activity and stretches can alleviate these issues.

MOVEMENT BREAKS

Deskbound workers spend an average of 75 per cent of their work hours sitting, often in prolonged and unbroken bouts of 30 minutes or more. It is suggested that neck and lower body pain is associated with prolonged sitting, and upper body issues can be aggravated with computer use.

It is important to take regular breaks during the working day to reduce sitting time. It is also advised to include physical activity, which may not only reduce pain; it could also improve focus, mood, memory, and more. Addressing the thoracic spine can help reduce neck pain, and general stretching can improve overall health.

Basic relaxation

Static stretches:
Hold 15–30 seconds

Dynamic stretches (D):
Do 10–15 reps at 1–2 second holds

---

1. Levator Stretch p.68

---

2. Manual Suboccipital Stretch p.69

---

3. Sternocleidomastoid Stretch p.70

---

4. Seated Cat Cow (D) p.75

---

5. Seated Quadratus Lumborum Stretch (D) p.77

---

6. Wrist Extension & Wrist Flexion Stretch p.108

---

7. Seated Figure 4 Stretch p.129

Daily stretch break

Static stretches:
Hold 15–30 seconds

Dynamic stretches (D):
Do 10–15 reps at 1–2 second holds

---

1. Standing Thoracic Extension Wall Stretch (D) p.84

---

2. Quadratus Lumborum Stretch (D) p.76

---

3. Standing Half Moon (D) p.92

---

4. Thread the Needle (D) p.94

---

5. Doorway Pec Stretch p.102

---

6. Chair/Elevated Hip Flexor Stretch p.137

---

7. Seated Hamstring Stretch p.162

ROUTINES FOR OLDER ADULTS

Aging skeletal muscle still maintains the ability to adapt. Older adults should strive to stay active; stretches offer a form of light-intensity movement to challenge coordination and neuromuscular control.

Stretches should supplement a well-rounded routine that includes balance, aerobic, and moderate-intensity resistance training (see p.54). Programmes can be tailored towards daily function and goals, like walking and engaging in enjoyable activities.

Physical activity in older adults can improve outcomes for cardiovascular disease, high blood pressure, type 2 diabetes, cognitive health, and sleep. It also reduces mortality risk. Exercise can also help prevent falls, fall-related injuries, and declines in bone health. Focus on stretching joints used in daily life, like the hips, trunk, and lower legs. Stretching the trunk muscles can increase spinal mobility, while stretching the hip flexors can improve gait. Try different types of stretches, and stay within a tolerable level of intensity. Some studies have found people under 65 years old respond better to PNF stretching (see p.42), whereas those over 65 may benefit more from static stretching (see p.41). Static stretches for older adults may need to be held for longer durations to impact flexibility.

> *Stretching routines for older adults can help maintain flexibility, improve mobility, and enhance overall physical wellbeing.*

Upper body focus

Static stretches:
Hold 20–60 seconds

Dynamic stretches (D):
Do 10–15 reps at 2–3 second holds

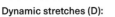

1. Seated Cat Cow (D) p.75

2. Seated Quadratus Lumborum Stretch (D) p.77

3. Cobra (variations) p.82

4. Standing Thoracic Rotation (D) p.90

5. Doorway Pec Stretch p.102

Lower body focus

Static stretches:
Hold 20–60 seconds

Dynamic stretches (D):
Do 10–15 reps at 2–3 second holds

1. Cross Body Glute Stretch p.130

2. Figure 4 Hip Internal Rotation Stretch (D) p.132

3. Standing Hip Flexor Stretch p.136

4. Bent-Knee Calf Stretch (hold each stage) p.168

5. Seated Hamstring Stretch p.162

ROUTINES FOR WALKERS

Walking is a simple and often accessible way to continue to stay active. The muscles of the hips, knees, and ankles are the most active in walking, and the demands on them vary based on different terrains and inclines.

You can reduce the risk of sustaining injuries when walking by following a few simple guidelines. Make sure you wear proper footwear, set goals, improve endurance and tolerance, warm up, listen to your body, and include a proper training programme in your schedule regularly.

LOWER BODY FOCUS

Walking uses various muscles in the body, especially those in the lower body. The hip flexors lift the leg to initiate the motion forward.

The quadriceps work to extend the knee joint in taking the first step. The tibialis anterior, in front of the shin, helps with ankle dorsiflexion to clear the foot as the leg comes forward. The hamstrings, behind the thigh, help to flex the knee and control the leg swing as it moves back during the walking motion.

The glutes, particularly the gluteus medius, are important for hip extension and keeping the pelvis level. They provide power during the push-off phase, as well as pelvic stability. The calves play a significant role in ankle plantarflexion, which propels the body forward during each step.

The tibialis anterior helps with ankle dorsiflexion to clear the foot as the leg comes forward. The specific contribution of these muscles can vary depending on factors like walking speed, incline, and individual biomechanics. However, if you warm up properly and keep these muscles flexible, you will be taking steps to maintain healthy walking ability throughout your lifespan.

Dynamic warmup

Dynamic stretches:
Do 10–15 reps at
1–2 second holds

1. Gastrocnemius Wall Stretch p.166

2. Gastrocnemius Step Stretch p.164

3. Seated Hamstring Stretch p.162

4. Standing Hip Circles p.148

5. Standing Hip Flexor Stretch p.136

6. Standing Half Moon p.92

7. Quadratus Lumborum Stretch p.76

Mobility beginner

Static stretches:
Hold 15–30 seconds
Dynamic stretches (D):
Do 10–15 reps at
1–2 second holds

1. Cat Cow (D) p.74

2. Cobra p. 80

3. Static Hamstring Stretch p.160

4. Cross Body Glute Stretch p.130

5. Half-Kneel Hip Flexor Stretch p.134

6. Quadruped Hip Circle (D) p.150

7. Standing Quad Stretch p.157

Mobility advanced

Static stretches:
Hold 15–30 seconds
Dynamic stretches (D):
Do 10–15 reps at
1–2 second holds

1. Quadratus Lumborum Stretch p.76

2. Half-kneel Thoracic Rotation p.88

3. Bretzel p.91

4. Dynamic Hamstring Lowers (D) p.163

5. Hamstring Rockback (D) p.121

6. Gastrocnemius Wall Stretch (D) p.166

7. Standing Hip Circles (D) p.148

ROUTINES FOR RUNNERS

Running involves a higher intensity and impact compared to walking, requiring a greater recruitment and coordination of muscles throughout the body. Work up to it by starting with walking and jogging combinations, gradually progressing.

Running is involved in many sports and is an activity itself. It is a complex movement that involves coordination and interaction among multiple muscle groups to generate power, maintain balance, and absorb impact forces.

REDUCING INJURY RISK
Proper strength training and conditioning of the lower body muscle groups can help improve running performance and reduce the risk of injuries. Other things to note include gradual programming of running distance, intensity, and duration, along with proper footwear. Keeping the muscles of the lower body prepared for the necessary run tasks is critical.

Muscles used include the hip flexors and extensors, knee extensors and flexors, and ankle plantarflexors. The quadriceps and glutes generate power and propel the body forward, while the hamstrings control leg swing and provide stability. The calves contribute to ankle propulsion and shock absorption.

80%
OF DISORDERS ARE **OVERUSE INJURIES,** A MISMATCH BETWEEN THE **RESILIENCE OF THE TISSUE** AND RUNNING

Dynamic warmup

Dynamic stretches:
Do 10–15 reps at
1–2 second holds

1. Gastrocnemius Wall Stretch p.166

2. Gastrocnemius Step Stretch p.164

3. World's Greatest Stretch p.140

4. Garland Squat p.126

5. Standing Hip Circles p.148

6. Half-Kneel Hip Flexor Rock p.122

7. Dynamic Hamstring Lowers p.163

Mobility beginner

Static stretches:
Hold 15–30 seconds
Dynamic stretches (D):
Do 10–15 reps at
1–2 second holds

1. Cat Cow (D) p.4

2. Standing Quad Stretch p.157

3. Static Hamstring Stretch p.160

4. Elevated Hip Flexor stretch p. 137

5. Gastrocnemius Wall Stretch p. 166 (D)

6. Quadruped Hip Circle (D) p.150

7. Dynamic Hamstring Lowers (D) p.163

Mobility advanced

Dynamic stretches:
Do 10–15 reps at
1–2 second holds

1. Ankle Dorsiflexion Rock p.169

2. Adductor Rockback p.120

3. Diagonal Flexor Rock p.124

4. Hamstring Rockback p. 121

5. Dynamic Hamstring Lowers p.163

6. Gastrocnemius Step Stretch p.164

7. Standing Hip Circles p.148

ROUTINES FOR CYCLISTS

Both cycling and stationary biking provide a low impact cardiovascular workout that primarily targets the lower body muscles. Stretching can help relieve tension in the muscles used most often and prepare them for activity.

The primary muscle groups recruited during cycling include the hip flexors, quadriceps, hamstrings, glutes, calves, and core muscles. Proper muscle coordination and activation are essential to achieve an efficient pedalling technique, generate power, and enhance overall cycling performance.

While cycling requires greater use of the upper body to maintain stability and control than a stationary cycle, similar muscle groups, including the core, are used in both activities. Strengthening and conditioning these muscle groups can improve cycling efficiency, endurance, and reduce the risk of overuse injuries. The quads help extend the knee during the downstroke of pedalling, while the hamstrings are involved in the upstroke phase and assist in flexing the knee. The hip flexors help lift the leg and drive the knee upward during the upstroke phase of the pedalling, aiding in a smooth pedal stroke. To maintain good mobility, target these muscle groups when you are training.

UP TO
17%
OF **INJURIES** AMONG **CYCLISTS** ARE REPORTED TO BE **MUSCLE** OR **TENDON** RELATED

Dynamic warmup

Dynamic stretches:
Do 10–15 reps at
1–2 second holds

1. Downward Dog Alternating Knee Bend p.169

2. Adductor Rockback p.120

3. World's Greatest Stretch p.140

4. Garland Squat p.126

5. Standing Hip Circles p. 148

6. Half-Kneel Hip Flexor Rock p.122

7. Hamstring Rockback p.121

Mobility beginner

Static stretches:
Hold 15–30 seconds
Dynamic stretches (D):
Do 10–15 reps at 1–2 second holds

1. Quadruped Rockback (D) p.114

2. Standing Thoracic Extension Wall Stretch p.84

3. Standing Quad Stretch p.157

4. Static Hamstring Stretch p.160

5. Standing Hip Flexor Stretch p.136

6. Cobra p.80

7. Quadruped Hip Circle (D) p.150

Mobility advanced

Static stretches:
Hold 15–30 seconds
Dynamic stretches(D):
Do 10–15 reps at 1–2 second holds

1. Half-Kneel Couch Stretch p.159

2. Adductor Rockback (D) p.120

3. Diagonal Hip Flexor Rock (D) p.124

4. Hamstring Rockback (D) p.121

5. Figure 4 Hip Internal Rotation Stretch (D) p.132

6. Gastrocnemius Step Stretch (D) p.164

7. Standing Hip Circles (D) p.148

ROUTINES FOR SWIMMERS

Swimming offers a low-impact, full-body workout that engages a range of both large and small muscle groups. It provides cardiovascular benefits while also developing muscular strength, endurance, and flexibility.

Swimming relies heavily on the muscles of the upper body, including the deltoids, pectorals, latissimus dorsi, scapular, and rotator cuff muscles. The core and back muscles help to maintain posture, stability, and propulsion during swimming.

Swimming requires a wide range of motion in the shoulders, hips, and other joints. Adequate flexibility allows swimmers to achieve the necessary arm and leg movements with optimal technique and efficiency. Flexibility is crucial for executing proper stroke techniques, enabling swimmers to achieve longer, more efficient strokes, and maintain body alignment. Having a flexible spine, hips, and shoulders allows swimmers to efficiently get in position for quick push-offs from swimming pool walls, and transitions during flip turns and dive starts. Including regular flexibility exercises in a swimmer's training routine can help improve range of motion, enhance stroke technique, and reduce the risk of swimming-related injuries.

Swimming works your entire body, including your heart and lungs, and can also boost your mood.

Dynamic warmup

Dynamic stretches:
Do 10–15 reps at
1–2 second holds

1. Frog Rockback p. 121

2. Standing Thoracic Extension Wall Stretch p.84

3. Quadratus Lumborum Stretch p.76

4. Twisted Cobra p. 81

5. Lateral Flexor Rock p.125

6. Figure 4 Hip Internal Rotation Stretch p.132

7. World's Greatest Stretch p.140

Mobility beginner

Static stretches:
Hold 15–30 seconds
Dynamic stretches (D):
Do 10–15 reps at 1–2 second holds

1. Frog Rockback (D) p.121

2. Adductor Rockback (D) p.120

3. Puppy Pose p.86

4. Cross Body Arm Stretch p.105

5. Floor Angel (D) p.106

6. Doorway Pec Stretch p.98

7. Cobra: Hands Far Away p.82

Mobility advanced

Static stretches:
Hold 15–30 seconds
Dynamic stretches (D):
Do 10–15 reps at 1–2 second holds

1. Mermaid (D) p.97

2. Thread the Needle in Adductor Stretch (D) p.96

3. Quadruped Hip Circle (D) p.150

4. Half-Kneel Couch Stretch p.159

5. Dynamic Hamstring Lowers (D) p.163

6. Gastrocnemius Step Stretch (D) p.164

7. Standing Thoracic Extension Wall Stretch (D) p.84

ROUTINES FOR STRENGTH TRAINING

Stretching to accompany a strength training routine can be done in a variety of ways. You can stretch as a standalone routine to train flexibility relevant to individual goals, or as part of a warmup or cool down.

Light-intensity stretching and strength training can each increase range of motion. With increases in range of motion, stretch intensities may need to be adjusted to continuously challenge the limits, which sometimes is not feasible with strength training if the person has not progressed their strength to do so yet. By combining stretching and strength training, one can achieve a well-rounded exercise routine that promotes strength, flexibility, and overall physical wellbeing.

MATCHING LIFTING DEMANDS
There are several classic exercises that are commonly found in gyms and are considered fundamental for strength training. These exercises target multiple muscle groups and provide a solid foundation for building strength and muscle mass. Squats, deadlifts, bench press, shoulder press, pull-ups, rows, lunges, and tricep extensions are a few common exercises that provide a solid foundation for full-body strength training. When choosing stretches to supplement strength training, select stretches that specifically target the muscle groups worked during the strength training session. For example, before deadlifts, opt for dynamic stretches for optimal performance. After deadlifts, use stretches for the hamstrings and lower back.

Dynamic warmup

Dynamic stretches:
Do 10–15 reps at
1–2 second holds

1. Dynamic Hamstring Lowers p.163

2. Adductor Rockback p.120

3. Garland Squat p.126

4. Thread the Needle p.94

5. Quadratus Lumborum Stretch p.76

6. Garland Squat: Alternating Arm Reach p.127

7. World's Greatest Stretch p.140

Mobility beginner

Static stretches:
Hold 15–30 seconds
Dynamic stretches (D):
Do 10–15 reps at
1–2 second holds

1. Thread the Needle: Hand Behind Head (D) p.96

2. Standing Thoracic Extension Wall Stretch (D) p. 84

3. Twisted Cobra p.81

4. Child's Pose: Lateral p.79

5. Cross Body Arm Stretch p.105

6. Floor Angels p. 106 (D)

7. Quadruped Hip Circle (D) p.150

Mobility advanced

Static stretches:
Hold 15–30 seconds
Dynamic stretches (D):
Do 10–15 reps at
1–2 second holds

1. Thoracic Stretch: Arms on a Chair (D) p. 86

2. Pigeon Stretch p.138

3. Thread the Needle in Adductor Stretch (D) p. 96

4. Half-Kneel Couch Stretch p.159

5. Standing Hip Circles (D) p.148

6. Bretzel p.91

7. Half-Kneel Thoracic Rotation (D) p.88

ROUTINES FOR ATHLETES

Several sports heavily emphasize lower body strength, power, and agility. Running, soccer, basketball, American football, track and field sports (such as hurdling), and even skiing require substantial effort from the lower body.

Depending on individual needs, stretches can be performed as shown in this book or tailored to match the sport, position, or type of athlete. For example, a dancer will choose to move into a greater range of motion during a stretch when preparing for a dance performance.

TRAINING PROGRAMMES

Stretching helps improve flexibility, which is crucial for runners and jumpers. Adequate flexibility in the lower body muscles, such as the calves, hamstrings, and hip flexors, allows for a longer and more efficient stride in running and a greater range of motion in jumping movements, such as clearing hurdles.

Prior to running or jumping activities, dynamic stretching is often more effective than static stretching for warming up the muscles. Dynamic stretches involve controlled movements that mimic the motions of the activity, such as leg swings or walking lunges. This type of stretching helps improve joint mobility, activates the muscles, and enhances neuromuscular coordination.

UP TO
55%
OF ALL MUSCLE INJURIES HAPPEN DURING SPORTS ACTIVITY

Dynamic warmup

Dynamic stretches:
Do 10–15 reps at 1–2 second holds

1. Thread the Needle in Adductor Stretch p.96

2. Adductor Rockback p.120

3. Hamstring Rockback p.121

4. Dynamic Hamstring Lowers p.163

5. Lateral Flexor Rock p.125

6. World's Greatest Stretch p.140

7. Gastrocnemius Wall Stretch p.166

Mobility beginner

Static stretches:
Hold 15–30 seconds
Dynamic stretches (D):
Do 10–15 reps at 1–2 second holds

1. Half-Kneel Thoracic Rotation p.88

2. Static Hamstring Stretch p.160

3. Garland Squat (D) p.126

4. Figure 4 Stretch p.128

5. Cross Body Glute Stretch p. 130

6. Frog Rockback (D) p.121

7. Half-Kneel Hip Flexor Stretch p.134

Mobility advanced

Static stretches:
Hold 15–30 seconds
Dynamic stretches (D):
Do 10–15 reps at 1–2 second holds

1. Bretzel p.91

2. Pigeon Stretch p.138

3. Gastrocnemius Step Stretch (D) p.164

4. Half-Kneel Couch Stretch p.159

5. Word's Greatest Stretch (D) p.140

6. Standing Hip Circles (D) p.148

7. Standing Hip Flexor Stretch p.134

ROUTINES FOR OVERHEAD/ RACQUET SPORTS

Overhead and racquet sports, such as tennis and volleyball, require extensive shoulder mobility and flexibility. Stretching the arms and wrists helps improve mobility and flexibility, allowing for more power and control in shots or swings.

In overhead and racquet sports, the primary muscle groups involved are the shoulder muscles (deltoids and rotator cuff), arm muscles (biceps and triceps), core muscles (abdominals and lower back), leg muscles (quadriceps and hamstrings), and wrist/hand muscles. These muscles generate power, provide stability, and control movements during overhead strokes or racquet swings. Strengthening and conditioning

these muscle groups contribute to improved performance and injury prevention in these sports.

MULTIPLANAR MOVEMENT

This refers to movement that occurs in multiple planes of motion (see p.14), namely the sagittal plane (forwards and backwards), frontal plane (side to side), and transverse plane (rotational). In overhead and racquet sports, multiplanar movement is highly relevant.

Strokes in these sports involve complex movement patterns that incorporate all three planes of motion. For example, a tennis serve requires forward arm extension (sagittal plane), torso rotation (transverse plane), and weight transfer (frontal plane). Multiplanar movement allows athletes to generate power, accuracy, and efficiency in their strokes. Target the muscles that perform these motions for mobility training.

Warmup

Static stretches:
Hold 15–30 seconds
Dynamic stretches (D):
Do 10-15 reps at 1-2 second holds

1. Standing Thoracic Extension Wall Stretch p. 84 (D)

2. Thread the Needle (D) p.94

3. Half-Kneel Thoracic Rotation (D) p.88

4. Diagonal Flexor Rock (D) p.124

5. Adductor Rockback (D) p.120

6. Wrist Extension & Wrist Flexion p.108

7. Pec Minor Stretch p.104

Mobility beginner

Static stretches:
Hold 15–30 seconds
Dynamic stretches (D):
Do 10–15 reps at 1–2 second holds

1. Standing Thoracic Rotation (D) p.90

2. Standing Half Moon (D) p.92

3. Doorway Pec Stretch p.98

4. Cross Body Arm Stretch p.105

5. Floor Angel (D) p.106

6. Cobra p.80

7. Standing Thoracic Extension Wall Stretch (D) p.84

Mobility advanced

Static stretches:
Hold 15–30 seconds
Dynamic stretches (D):
Do 10–15 reps at 1–2 second holds

1. World's Greatest Stretch (D) p.140

2. Thread the Needle in Adductor Stretch (D) p.96

3. Standing Hip Circle (D) p.148

4. Child's Pose: Lateral p.79

5. Bretzel p.91

6. Gastrocnemius Step Stretch (D) p.164

7. Twisted Cobra p.81

ROUTINES FOR MARTIAL ARTS PRACTITIONERS

Martial arts require a wide range of motion and flexibility. Stretching exercises help improve flexibility, allowing martial artists to perform high kicks, deep stances, and fluid movements with greater ease and reduced risk of injury.

Stretching exercises that target the core muscles, such as the abdominal and back muscles, contribute to improved balance and stability in martial arts. This enhances the ability to maintain strong stances, execute precise movements, and resist opponents' attacks. Stretching can also help increase the flexibility of the hip flexors, hamstrings, and calf muscles, enabling those practising martial arts to achieve higher kicks, better extension, and improved kicking technique.

WHAT MUSCLES ARE USED?

Martial arts often involve high kicks, swift footwork, and dynamic lower body movements. Adequate leg flexibility is essential for achieving high kicks, executing quick and powerful kicks with proper form, and maintaining balance during kicks and stances. It involves flexibility in the hip flexors, hamstrings, quadriceps, and calf muscles. Having good hip and pelvic mobility allows for fluid transitions between techniques, facilitates effective grappling and takedown manoeuvres, and enhances overall agility. A supple spine is beneficial in martial arts, particularly in disciplines that involve throws, ground fighting, and evasive manoeuvres. Upper body flexibility also aids in grappling and defence techniques.

Dynamic warmup

Dynamic stretches:
Do 10–15 reps at 1–2 second holds

1. Garland Squat p.126

2. Adductor Rockback p.120

3. Hamstring Rockback p.121

4. Half-Kneel Hip Flexor Rock p.123

5. Lateral Flexor Rock p.125

6. Figure 4 Hip Internal Rotation Stretch p.132

7. World's Greatest Stretch p.140

Mobility beginner

Static stretches:
Hold 15–30 seconds
Dynamic stretches (D):
Do 10–15 reps at 1–2 second holds

1. Frog Rockback (D) p.121

2. Puppy Pose p.86

3. Cobra p.80

4. Floor Angel (D) p.106

5. Doorway Pec Stretch p.98

6. Bretzel p.91

7. Child's Pose p.78

Mobility advanced

Dynamic stretches:
Do 10–15 reps at 1–2 second holds

1. Mermaid p.97

2. Floor Wrist Extension & Flexion p.110

3. Thread the Needle in Adductor Stretch p.96

4. Quadruped Hip Circle p.150

5. Dynamic Hamstring Lowers p.163

6. Standing Thoracic Extension Wall Stretch p. 84

7. Word's Greatest Stretch p.140

GLOSSARY

Abduction The motion of a limb away from the body's midline.

Active tension The force created by the interactions of the myofibrils in a working muscle.

Adduction The motion of a limb or body segment towards the body's midline.

Anterior The front or front-facing structure of the body, also called "ventral".

Central sensitization A heightened nervous system response resulting in increased pain or hypersensitivity to stimuli: 'centralized pain".

Cervical The region of the spine located in the neck.

Concentric contraction The act of a muscle length shortening during contraction: the "positive" contraction.

Contractility A muscle's ability to generate active tension.

Coronal plane Oriented vertically to divide the body into anterior and posterior parts.

Distal Describes something further from the structure's origin.

Dorsiflexion An ankle joint motion that points the foot towards the shin, decreasing the angle between the foot and leg.

Eccentric contraction The act of muscle length lengthening during contraction: the "negative" contraction.

Elasticity The ability of a muscle to return to its original length when relaxed.

Eversion An outward motion at the foot and ankle that turns the sole away from body's midline.

Excitability A muscle's ability to respond to a stimulus, such as a motor neuron.

Extensibility The ability of a muscle and other connective tissue elements to elongate.

Extension A joint motion that increases the angle between two body parts.

External rotation A rotational joint motion away from body's midline; also known as medial rotation.

Fascia The connective tissue sheath that separates, surrounds, and supports organs, muscles, nerves, and other bodily structures.

Femoral nerve A nerve located in the thigh that supplies sensation to the front of the thigh and inner leg, as well as controlling certain muscles in the leg, including the quadriceps.

Fibular nerve A branch of the sciatic nerve in the lower leg that provides feeling to the top of the foot and controls some of the muscles involved in moving the foot and ankle; also referred to as the peroneal nerve.

Flexibility The ability a muscle has to lengthen and allow a joint, or joints, to move through a range of motion.

Flexion A joint motion that decreases the angle between two body parts.

Force The muscle fibres' active tension, or strength of the muscular contraction.

Golgi tendon organ (GTO) Sensory receptor in a muscle-tendon junction detecting tension, inhibiting excessive force, and protecting muscle-tendon integrity.

Inferior The position of something deeper and further from the surface of the body.

Internal rotation A rotational joint motion towards the body's midline, also known as medial rotation.

Inversion An inward motion at the foot and ankle that turns the sole towards the body's midline.

Isometric A muscle contraction without a change in muscle length or joint motion.

Kyphosis A natural outward curvature of the spine, commonly seen in the upper back (thoracic region)

Lateral A position or structure that is further from the midline of the body.

Lordosis A natural inward curvature of the spine, typically observed in the region of the lower back (lumbar region) or neck (cervical region).

Lumbar The region of the spine located in the lower back.

Medial A position or structure that is close to the midline of the body.

Median nerve A major nerve in the arm that provides sensory and motor function to the forearm, wrist, and hand.

Mobility The capacity to move efficiently, without limitations or restrictions, with adequate flexibility, stability, and motor control, within a joint or through a movement pattern.

Motor cortex The part of the brain's frontal lobe involved in planning, controlling, and executing voluntary movement.

Muscle spindle A specialized sensory receptor located within the muscle that detects changes, and speed of change, in muscle length.

Myofibril Larger organelles (small structures in a cell) composed of bundled myofilaments.

Myofilaments The thick and thin protein filaments that are responsible for muscle contraction.

Neurodynamics The interaction between the nervous system, and nerves and their movement, in relation to the musculoskeletal system.

Neurogenesis The process through with new neurons are formed in the brain.

Osteoarthritis A common and multifaceted disorder of the joints characterized by inflammation, pain, stiffness, and changes within the joint.

Pain An unpleasant sensory and emotional experience associated with, or resembling, that associated with actual or potential tissue damage.

Passive tension The force created by elongating the connective tissue elements in a muscle-tendon unit.

Pelvic floor A group of muscles that span the bottom of the pelvis and support the pelvic organs.

Plantarflexion An ankle joint motion that points the foot away from shin, increasing the angle between the foot and leg.

Posterior The front or back-facing structure of the body, also called "ventral".

Prone A position in which the body is lying face down.

Proximal Something closer to the structure's origin.

Quadruped A position on the hands and knees; can also be called "all fours".

Radial nerve A major nerve in the upper limb that provides sensory and motor function to part of the triceps, forearm muscles, and hand.

Range of motion The degree of movement that occurs at a joint.

Rotator cuff A a group of muscles that control and stabilize the shoulder joint, including the teres minor, infraspinatus, subscapularis, and supraspinatus.

Sagittal plane Oriented vertically and perpendicular to the coronal plane, dividing the body into right and left parts.

Sarcopenia A syndrome characterized by progressive and generalized loss of skeletal muscle mass and strength, commonly associated with older adults.

Scapular muscles A term referring to muscles responsible for moving and stabilizing the scapula, including the levator scapulae, trapezius, rhomboids, and serratus anterior.

Sciatic nerve The largest nerve in the body, that originates in the lower back and travels down the back of the thigh, supplying the muscles and skin of the leg and foot.

Stability The ability to control the position or motion at a joint, influenced by dynamic (neuromuscular) and static (non-contractile) elements.

Stretching A movement applied by an external or internal force in order to increase one's joint range of motion.

Suboccipital (region) The area of the head just below the base of the skull.

Superior The position of something that is closer to the surface of the body.

Supine A position in which the body is lying face up.

Sural nerve A branch of the sciatic nerve that travels along the back of the lower leg, providing sensation to the outer side of the foot, and part of the calf.

Synovial joint A freely mobile joint in the body characterized by its joint cavity, and surrounded by an art icular capsule

Temporal (region) Side area of the head that is located on each side, extending from the temple to the top of the ear and the upper part of the cheekbone.

Thoracic The region of the spine located in the upper and middle back.

Tibial nerve A branch of the sciatic nerve situated in the lower leg that provides sensation to the sole of the foot and controls several muscles involved in foot movement and stability.

Transverse plane Divides the body into superior and inferior parts, also known as the horizontal or axial plane.

Ulnar nerve A major nerve in the arm that provides sensory and motor function to the medial forearm, wrist, and fourth and fifth fingers.

Vertebrae The individual bones that make up the spine.

INDEX

BIBLIOGRAPHY

8–9 Introduction (myths)

Herbert R.D., de Noronha M., Kamper S.J., "Stretching to prevent or reduce muscle soreness after exercise", Cochrane Database Syst Rev. 2011 Jul 6;(7):CD004577. doi: 10.1002/14651858.CD004577.pub3. PMID: 21735398.

Andersen J.C., "Stretching before and after exercise: effect on muscle soreness and injury risk", *J Athl Train*, 2005 Jul–Sep;40(3):218-20. PMID: 16284645; PMCID: PMC1250267.

Afonso J., Clemente F.M., Nakamura F.Y., Morouço P., Sarmento H., Inman R.A., Ramirez-Campillo R., "The Effectiveness of Post-exercise Stretching in Short-Term and Delayed Recovery of Strength, Range of Motion and Delayed Onset Muscle Soreness: A Systematic Review and Meta-Analysis of "Randomized Controlled Trials", *Front Physiol.*, 2021 May 5;12:67758. doi: 10.3389/fphys.2021.677581. PMID: 34025459; PMCID: PMC8133317.

12–13: Anatomy of Movement

Schwartz A. B., "Movement: How the Brain Communicates with the World", *Cell*, 2016 Mar 10;164(6):1122–1135. doi: 10.1016/j.cell.2016.02.038. PMID: 26967280; PMCID: PMC4818644.

Gadhvi M., Waseem M., "Physiology, Sensory System", [Updated 2022 May 8]. In: StatPearls[Internet]. Treasure Island (FL): StatPearls Publishing; 2023 Jan-. Available from: https://www.ncbi.nlm.nih.gov/books/NBK547656/.

Dean J. C., "Proprioceptive feedback and preferred patterns of human movement", *Exerc Sport Sci Rev,* 2013 Jan, 41(1):36-43. doi: 10.1097/JES.0b013e3182724bb0. PMID: 23038242; PMCID: PMC5997460.

Panidi, I., Bogdanis, G. C., Terzis, G., et al. (2021), "Muscle Architectural and Functional Adaptations Following 12-Weeks of Stretching in Adolescent Female Athletes", *Frontiers in Physiology,* vol. 12, article 701338.

Nakamura, M. et al. (2020), "Effects of Static Stretching Programs Performed at Different Volume-Equated Weekly Frequencies on Passive Properties of Muscle-Tendon Unit", *Journal of Biomechanics,* vol. 103, article 109670.

Freitas S. R, Mendes B., Le Sant G., Andrade R.J., Nordez A.,

Milanovic Z., "Can chronic stretching change the muscle-tendon mechanical properties? A review", *Scand J Med Sci Sports*, 2018 Mar;28(3):794-806. doi: 10.1111/sms.12957. Epub 2017 Oct 9. PMID: 28801950.

18–19: Muscle Chains and Groupings

Lee, D., Vleeming, A., Jones, M.,*The Pelvic Girdle: An Integration of Clinical Expertise and Research*, Edinburgh: Elsevier/Churchill Livingstone, 2011.

Bordoni B., Myers T. A .,"Review of the Theoretical Fascial Models: Biotensegrity, Fascintegrity, and Myofascial Chains", *Cureus*, 2020 Feb 24;12(2):e7092. doi: 10.7759/cureus.7092. PMID: 32226693; PMCID: PMC7096016.

Wilke J., Krause F., Vogt L., Banzer W., "What Is Evidence-Based About Myofascial Chains: A Systematic Review", *Arch Phys Med Rehabil*, 2016 Mar;97(3):454-61. doi: 10.1016/j.apmr.2015.07.023. Epub 2015 Aug 14. PMID: 26281953.

Bergmark A., "Stability of the lumbar spine. A study in mechanical engineering", *Acta Orthop Scand Suppl,* 1989;230:1-54. doi: 10.3109/17453678909154177. PMID: 2658468.

20–21: How Muscles Work

Lieber, R. L. (2002) *Skeletal Muscle Structure, Function, and Plasticity*, Lippincott Williams & Wilkins, Philadelphia.

Robbins, Dan, Chapter 7 Muscle Biomechanics in: Innocenti, B. Galbusera, F. (2022) *Human Orthopaedic Biomechanics*, Academic Press. 1st Edition, pp. 121–135.

O'Sullivan, K., McAuliffe, S., DeBurca, N. (2012), "The Effects of Eccentric Training on Lower Limb Flexibility: A Systematic Review", *British Journal of Sports Medicine,* vol. 46, no. 12, pp. 833–834.

Baechle, T. R., & Earle, R. W. (2008), *Essentials of strength training and conditioning*, 3rd ed. Champaign, IL, Human Kinetics.

Dougas, J., Pearson, S., Ross, A., McGuidan, M. (2017), "Chronic Adaptations to Eccentric Training: A Systematic Review", *Sports Medicine,* vol. 47, no. 917–941.

22–23: Anatomy of a Muscle

McMahon, T. A. (1984), *Muscles, Reflexes, and Locomotion*, Princeton University Press, New Jersey.

26–27: Skeletal System: Spine and Pelvis

Kim D., Davis D. D., Menger R. P., "Spine Sagittal Balance", [Updated 2022 Aug 8]. In: StatPearls[Internet]. Treasure Island (FL): StatPearls Publishing; 2023 Jan-. Available from: https://www.ncbi.nlm.nih.gov/books/NBK534858/

Herrington L., "Assessment of the degree of pelvic tilt within a normal asymptomatic population", *Man Ther.*, 2011 Dec;16(6):646–8. doi: 10.1016/j.math.2011.04.006. Epub 2011 Jun 11. PMID: 21658988.

Suits W. H., "Clinical Measures of Pelvic Tilt in Physical Therapy", *Int J Sports Phys Ther.*, 2021 Oct 1,16(5):1366-1375. doi: 10.26603/001c.27978. PMID: 34631258; PMCID: PMC8486407.

28–29: Joints

Luan L., El-Ansary D., Adams R., Wu S., Han J., "Knee osteoarthritis pain and stretching exercises: a systematic review and meta-analysis", *Physiotherapy*, 2022 Mar;114:16-29. doi: 10.1016/j.physio.2021.10.001. Epub 2021 Oct 11. PMID: 35091326.

30–31: Nervous System

Ellis R.F., Hing W. A., "Neural mobilization: a systematic review of randomized controlled trials with an analysis of therapeutic efficacy", *J Man Manip Ther.* 2008,16(1):8-22. doi: 10.1179/106698108790818594. PMID: 19119380; PMCID: PMC2565076.

Shacklock M. O., *Clinical Neurodynamics: A New System of Neuromusculoskeletal Treatment*, Oxford, UK: Butterworth Heinemann; 2005.

32–33: Nature and Theories of Pain

Raja, Srinivasa N. A., Carr, Daniel B. B, Cohen, Miltonc, Finnerup, Nanna B. D. E., Flor, Hertaf, Gibson, Stepheng, Keefe, Francis J. H., Mogil, Jeffrey S. I, Ringkamp, Matthias J., Sluka,

Kathleen A. K., Song, Xue-Junl, Stevens, Bonniem, Sullivan, Mark D. N.,Tutelman, Perri R. O., Ushida, Takahirop, Vader, Kyleq, "The revised International Association for the Study of Pain definition of pain: concepts, challenges, and compromises", *PAIN,* 161(9):p 1976–1982, September 2020. | DOI: 10.1097/j.pain.0000000000001939.

Smart K.M., Blake C., Staines A., Thacker M., Doody C., "Mechanisms-based classifications of musculoskeletal pain: part 1 of 3: symptoms and signs of central sensitisation in patients with low back (± leg) pain", *Man Ther.,* 2012 Aug;17(4):336–44.

El-Tallawy S. N., Nalamasu R., Salem G. I., LeQuang J. A. K., Pergolizzi JV, Christo P.J., "Management of Musculoskeletal Pain: An Update with Emphasis on Chronic Musculoskeletal Pain", *Pain Ther.,* 2021 Jun;10(1):181-209. doi: 10.1007/s40122-021–00235-2. Epub 2021 Feb 11. PMID: 33575952; PMCID: PMC8119532.

Lima L. V., Abner T. S. S., Sluka K.A., "Does exercise increase or decrease pain? Central mechanisms underlying these two phenomena", *J Physiol.,* 2017 Jul 1;595(13):4141-4150. doi: 10.1113/JP273355. Epub 2017 May 26. PMID: 28369946; PMCID: PMC5491894.

Yam M. F., Loh Y. C., Tan C. S., Khadijah Adam S., Abdul Manan N., Basir R., "General Pathways of Pain Sensation and the Major Neurotransmitters Involved in Pain Regulation", *Int J Mol Sci,.* 2018 Jul 24;19(8):2164. doi: 10.3390/ijms19082164. PMID: 30042373; PMCID: PMC6121522.

Bonezzi C., Fornasari D., Cricelli C., Magni A., Ventriglia G., "Not All Pain is Created Equal: Basic Definitions and Diagnostic Work-Up", *Pain Ther.,* 2020 Dec;9(Suppl 1):1-15. doi: 10.1007/s40122-020-00217-w. Epub 2020 Dec 14. PMID: 33315206; PMCID: PMC7736598.

Moseley, Lorimer (2007), "Reconceptualising pain according to modern pain science", *Physical Therapy Reviews,* 12. 169–178.

34–35: Movement and Brain Gains

Cotman, C. W., & Berchtold, N. C. (2002), "Exercise: a behavioral intervention to enhance brain health and plasticity", *Trends in Neurosciences*, 25(6), 295–301.

Erickson, K. I., Voss, M. W., Prakash, R. S., Basak, C., Szabo, A., Chaddock, L., Colcombe, S. J. (2011), "Exercise training increases size of hippocampus and improves memory", *Proceedings of the National Academy of Sciences*, 108(7), 3017–3022.

Varma V. R., Chuang Y.F., Harris G.C., Tan E.J., Carlson M.C., "Low-intensity daily walking activity is associated with hippocampal volume in older adults", *Hippocampus*, 2015 May;25(5):605-15. doi: 10.1002/hipo.22397. Epub 2014 Dec 26. PMID: 25483019; PMCID: PMC4425252.

36–39: Range of Motion and Flexibility

Diong J., Carden P.C., O'Sullivan K., Sherrington C., Reed D.S., "Eccentric exercise improves joint flexibility in adults: A systematic review update and meta-analysis", *Musculoskelet Sci Pract.*, 2022 Aug;60:102556. doi: 10.1016/j. msksp.2022.102556. Epub 2022 Mar 25. PMID: 35390669.

Apostolopoulos N., Metsios G. S., Flouris A. D., Koutedakis Y., Wyon M.A., "The relevance of stretch intensity and position – a systematic review.", *Front Psychol.*, 2015 Aug 18;6:1128. doi: 10.3389/fpsyg.2015.01128. PMID: 26347668; PMCID: PMC4540085.

Reddy, R. S. & Alahmari, K. A. (2016), "Effect of Lower Extremity Stretching Exercises on Balance in Geriatric Populations" *International Journal of Health Sciences,* vol. 10, no. 3, pp. 389–395.

Hasarangi, L. B. S. & Jayawardana, D. G. S K. (2018), "Comparison of Hamstring Flexibility Between Patients with Chronic Lower Back Pain and the Healthy Individuals at the National Hospital of Sri Lanka", *Biomedical Journal of Scientific & Technical Research,* vol. 5, no. 2.

Daylor, Victoria B .F. A.; Gensemer, Cortney PhD; Norris, Russell A. PhD, Bluestein, Linda MD, "Hope for Hypermobility: Part 1—An Integrative Approach to Treating Symptomatic Joint Hypermobility", *Topics in Pain Management,* 38(8):p 1–9, March 2023. | DOI: 10.1097/01.TPM.0000924780.91929.b3.

40–43: Types of Stretching

Page, P., "Current concepts in muscle stretching for exercise and rehabilitation", *Int J Sports Phys Ther.*,2012 Feb;7(1):109-19. PMID: 22319684; PMCID: PMC3273886.

Woolstenhulme M. T., Griffiths C. M., Woolstenhulme E. M., Parcell A. C., "Ballistic stretching increases flexibility and acute vertical jump height when combined with basketball activity", *J Strength Cond Res*, 2006 Nov;20(4):799–803. doi: 10.1519/R-18835.1. PMID: 17194248.

Mahieu N.N., McNair P., De Muynck M., Stevens V., Blanckaert I., Smits N., Witvrouw E., "Effect of static and ballistic stretching on the muscle-tendon tissue properties", *Med Sci Sports Exerc.,* 2007 Mar;39(3):494–501. doi: 10.1249/01. mss.0000247004.40212.f7. PMID: 17473776.

Iwata M., Yamamoto A., Matsuo S., Hatano G., Miyazaki M., Fukaya T., Fujiwara M., Asai Y., Suzuki S., "Dynamic Stretching Has Sustained Effects on Range of Motion and Passive Stiffness of the Hamstring Muscles", *J Sports Sci Med.*, 2019 Feb 11;18(1):13–20. PMID: 30787647; PMCID: PMC6370952.

Behm D. G., Blazevich A. J., Kay A. D., McHugh M., "Acute effects of muscle stretching on physical performance, range of motion, and injury incidence in healthy active individuals: a systematic review", *Appl Physiol Nutr Metab.*, 2016 Jan;41(1):1-11. doi: 10.1139/apnm-2015-0235. Epub2015 Dec 8. PMID: 26642915.Training Versus Stretching for Improving Range of Motion: A

Systematic Review and Meta-Analysis", *Healthcare*, volume 9, number 4, article 427.

Alizadeh, S., Daneshjoo, A., Zahiri, A., et al. (2023.) "Resistance Training Induces Improvements in Range of Motion: A Systematic Review and Meta-Analysis", *Sports Medicine*, epub ahead of print.

Hindle K. B., Whitcomb T. J., Briggs W. O., Hong J., "Proprioceptive Neuromuscular Facilitation (PNF): Its Mechanisms and Effects on Range of Motion and Muscular Function", *J Hum Kinet*, 2012 Mar;31:105-13. doi: 10.2478/v10078-012-0011-y. Epub 2012 Apr 3. PMID: 23487249; PMCID: PMC3588663.

44–47: Effects and Benefits of Stretching

Hotta K, Muller-Delp J., "Microvascular Adaptations to Muscle Stretch: Findings From Animals and the Elderly", *Front Physiol.*, 2022 Jul 4;13:939459. doi: 10.3389/fphys.2022.939459. PMID: 35860661; PMCID: PMC9289226.

Shariat A., Cleland J.A., Danaee M., Kargarfard M., Sangelaji B., Tamrin S. B. M., "Effects of stretching exercise training and ergonomic modifications on musculoskeletal discomforts of office workers: a randomized controlled trial", *Braz J Phys Ther.*, 2018 Mar–Apr;22(2):144–153. doi: 10.1016/j.bjpt.2017.09.003.

Epub 2017 Sep 6. PMID: 28939263; PMCID: PMC5883995.

Vecchio L. M., Meng Y., Xhima K., Lipsman N., Hamani C., Aubert I., "The Neuroprotective Effects of Exercise: Maintaining a Healthy Brain Throughout Aging", *Brain Plast.*, 2018 Dec 12;4(1):17–52. doi: 10.3233/BPL-180069. PMID: 30564545; PMCID: PMC6296262.

Thomas E., Bellafiore M., Petrigna L., Paoli A., Palma A., Bianco A., "Peripheral Nerve Responses to Muscle Stretching: A Systematic Review", *J Sports Sci Med.*, 2021 Mar 8;20(2):258-267. doi: 10.52082/jssm.2021.258. PMID: 34211318; PMCID: PMC8219270.

Sudo, Mizuki & Ando, Soichi (2019), "Effects of Acute Stretching on Cognitive Function and Mood States of Physically Inactive Young Adults", *Perceptual and Motor Skills*, 127. 10.1177/0031512519888304.

Pa J., Goodson W., Bloch A., King A. C., Yaffe K., Barnes D.E., "Effect of exercise and cognitive activity on self-reported sleep quality in community-dwelling older adults with cognitive complaints: a randomized controlled trial", *J Am GeriatrSoc.*, 2014 Dec;62(12):2319–26. doi: 10.1111/jgs.13158. PMID: 25516028; PMCID: PMC4356237.

Wipfli, B., Landers D., Nagoshi C., Ringenbach, S. (2011), "An examination of serotonin and psychological variables in the relationship between exercise and mental health", *Scandinavian Journal of Medicine & Science in Sports*, 21: 474–481. https://doi.org/10.1111/j.1600-0838.2009.01049.x

Ko J., Deprez D., Shaw K., Alcorn J., Hadjistavropoulos T., Tomczak C., Foulds H., Chilibeck P. D., "Stretching is Superior to Brisk Walking for Reducing Blood Pressure in People With High-Normal Blood Pressure or Stage I Hypertension", *J Phys Act Health*, 2021 Jan 1;18(1):21–28. doi: 10.1123/jpah.2020-0365. Epub 2020 Dec 18. Erratum in: J Phys Act Health. 2021 Apr 1;18(4):469. PMID: 33338988.

Otsuki T., Takanami Y., Aoi W., Kawai Y., Ichikawa, H., Yoshikawa T., Miyachi, M. (2008), "Arterial stiffness acutely decreases after whole-body passive stretching in hypertensive individuals", *European Journal of Applied Physiology*, 104(2), 228–235.

Nakamura M., Ikezoe T., Takeno Y., Ichihashi N., Kozakai, R. (2012), "Acute and prolonged effect of static stretching on the passive stiffness of the human gastrocnemius muscle tendon unit in vivo.", *Journal of Orthopaedic Research*, 30(3), 309–313.

48–48: Stretching and Maintaining Fitness

American College of Sports Medicine. (2018), *ACSM's guidelines for exercise testing and prescription*, Lippincott Williams & Wilkins.

McHugh, M. P., & Cosgrave, C. H. (2010), "To stretch or not to stretch: the role of stretching in injury prevention and performance", *Scandinavian Journal of Medicine & Science in Sports*, 20(2), 169–181.

ACSM (2009), American College of Sports Medicine position stand, "Progression models in resistance training for healthy adults", *Medicine & Science in Sports & Exercise*, 41(3), 687-708.

Nelson R. T., Bandy W. D., "Eccentric Training and Static Stretching Improve Hamstring Flexibility of High School Males", *J Athl Train.*, 2004 Sep;39(3):254–258. PMID: 15496995; PMCID: PMC522148.

50–53: Stretching for Injury Recovery and Pain Relief

Bahr R., Krosshaug T., "Understanding injury mechanisms: a key component of preventing injuries in sport", *British Journal of Sports Medicine,* 2005;39:324-329.

McHugh M. P., Cosgrave C. H., "To stretch or not to stretch: the role of stretching in injury prevention and performance", *Scandinavian Journal of Medicine & Science in Sports*, 2010 Apr;20(2):169–81. doi: 10.1111/j.1600-0838.2009.01058.x. Epub 2009 Dec 18. PMID: 20030776.

Witvrouw E, Mahieu N, Danneels L, McNair P., "Stretching and injury prevention: an obscure relationship", *Sports Med.*, 2004;34(7):443–9. doi: 10.2165/00007256-200434070-00003. PMID: 15233597.

Witvrouw E., Mahieu N., Roosen P., McNair P., "The role of stretching in tendon injuries", *British Journal of Sports Medicine*, 2007 Apr;41(4):224–6. doi: 10.1136/bjsm.2006.034165. Epub 2007 Jan 29. PMID: 17261561; PMCID: PMC2658965.

Geneen, L. J., Moore, R. A., Clarke, C., Martin, D., Colvin, L. A., & Smith, B. H. (2017), "Physical activity and exercise for chronic pain in adults: an overview of Cochrane Reviews", *Journal of Pain Research*, 10, 381–387.

Zeidan, F., Gordon, N. S., Merchant, J., & Goolkasian, P. (2010). "The effects of brief mindfulness meditation training on experimentally induced pain", *The Journal of Pain*, 11(3), 199-209.

Zeidan, F., Grant, J. A., Brown, C. A., McHaffie, J. G., & Coghill, R.

C. (2012). "Mindfulness meditation-related pain relief: Evidence for unique brain mechanisms in the regulation of pain", *Neuroscience Letters*, 520(2), 165–173.

Morone, N. E., Lynch, C. S., Greco, C. M., Tindle, H. A., & Weiner, D. K. (2008). "'I felt like a new person.' The effects of mindfulness meditation on older adults with chronic pain: Qualitative narrative analysis of diary entries", *Journal of Gerontological Nursing*, 34(4), 20–27.

Wiese-Bjornstal, D. M. (2009). "Sport Injury and College Athlete Health across the Lifespan", *Journal of Intercollegiate Sport*, 2(1), 64–80. https://doi.org/10.1123/jis.2.1.64

Dubois B., Esculier J., "Soft-tissue injuries simply need PEACE and LOVE", *British Journal of Sports Medicine* 2020;54:72–73.

Wang Z. R., Ni G. X., "Is it time to put traditional cold therapy in rehabilitation of soft-tissue injuries out to pasture?", *World J Clin Cases,* 2021 Jun 16;9(17):4116–4122. doi: 10.12998/wjcc. v9.i17.4116. PMID: 34141774; PMCID: PMC8173427.

54–57: Stretching and Healthy Aging

McCormick, R., Vasilaki, A., "Age-related changes in skeletal muscle: changes to life-style as a therapy", *Biogerontology*, 19, 519–536 (2018). https://doi.org/10.1007/s10522-018-9775-3.

Rider R. A., Daly J., "Effects of flexibility training on enhancing spinal mobility in older women", *J Sports Med Phys Fitness*, Jun 1991;31(2):213–217.

Rodacki A. L., Souza R. M., Ugrinowitsch C., Cristopoliski F., Fowler N. E., "Transient effects of stretching exercises on gait parameters of elderly women", *Man Ther.*, Apr 2009;14(2):167–172

Feland J. B., Myrer J. W., Schulthies S. S., Fellingham G. W., Measom G. W., "The effect of duration of stretching of the hamstring muscle group for increasing range of motion in people aged 65 years or older.", *Phys Ther*, May 2001;81(5):1110–1117

Page P., "Current concepts in muscle stretching for exercise and rehabilitation", *Int J Sports Phys Ther.*, 2012 Feb;7(1):109-19. PMID: 22319684; PMCID: PMC3273886.

58–59: When Not to Stretch

Hip joint variations: Pun, S., Kumar, D., Lane, N. E., Villar, R. N. (2016), "Hip morphology in the Asian population with and without developmental dysplasia", *The bone & joint journal,* 98-B(2), 202–207.

Ankle and hindfoot variations: Sailer, J., Margetić, P., Margetić, B. (2019), "Anatomical variation in the ankle and foot: from incidental finding to inductor of pathology. Part I: ankle and hindfoot", *Skeletal radiology*, 48(10), 1487–1498.

Knee joint variations: Qi, X. Z., & Xu, Z. J. (2020), "Association Between the Morphology of Proximal Tibiofibular Joint and the Presence of Knee OA", *Orthopaedic surgery*, 12(2), 503–510.

190–191: Introduction to the Routines

Opplert J., Babault N., "Acute Effects of Dynamic Stretching on Muscle Flexibility and Performance: An Analysis of the Current Literature", *Sports Med.*, 2018 Feb;48(2):299–325. doi: 10.1007/s40279-017-0797-9. PMID: 29063454.

Takeuchi K., Nakamura M., Matsuo S., Akizuki K., Mizuno T., "Effects of Speed and Amplitude of Dynamic Stretching on the Flexibility and Strength of the Hamstrings", *J Sports Sci Med.*, 2022 Dec 1;21(4):608-615. doi: 10.52082/jssm.2022.608. PMID: 36523896; PMCID: PMC9741718.

198: Routines for Deskbound Workers

Louw S., Makwela S., Manas L., Meyer L., Terblanche D., Brink Y., "Effectiveness of exercise in office workers with neck pain: A systematic review and meta-analysis", *S Afr J Physiother*, 2017 Nov 28;73(1):392. doi: 10.4102/sajp.v73i1.392. PMID: 30135909; PMCID: PMC6093121.

201: Routines for Runners

van der Worp M. P., ten Haaf D.S., van Cingel R., de Wijer A., Nijhuis-van der Sanden M.W., StaalJB, "Injuries in runners; a systematic review on risk factors and sex differences", *PLoS One,* 2015 Feb 23;10(2):e0114937. doi: 10.1371/journal. pone.0114937. PMID: 25706955; PMCID: PMC4338213.

202: Routines for Cyclists

Rooney D., Sarriegui I., Heron N., "'As easy as riding a bike': a systematic review of injuries and illness in road cycling", *BMJ Open Sport Exerc Med.*, 2020 Dec 9;6(1):e000840. doi: 10.1136/bmjsem-2020-000840. PMID: 34422283; PMCID: PMC8323466.

ABOUT THE AUTHOR

Dr Leada Malek, PT, DPT, CSCS, SCS, is a Doctor of Physical Therapy and board-certified sports clinical specialist. She is an NSCA Certified Strength and Conditioning Specialist and has taught DPT students as an Adjunct Faculty Instructor. She believes that mental and physical health are equally important, and this drives her passion for promoting exercise as a lifestyle for health and longevity. Dr. Malek's expertise has been featured in major publications such as Oxygen, Women's Health, Shape, and U.S. News. She has a strong social media presence where she shares her knowledge with thousands.

With extensive experience working with athletes at all levels, including professionals in sports and dance, Dr. Malek understands the complexities of the human body and power of movement as medicine. She has the ability to break down complex topics into digestible information and empower individuals through their movement journeys. When she's not treating or educating, Dr. Malek enjoys spending time with loved ones, exploring new restaurants, travelling, and listening to live music.

Connect with Dr Malek on Instagram **@drmalekpt** or visit **www.drmalekpt.com** to learn more.

ACKNOWLEDGEMENTS

Author acknowledgements

Writing this book was one of the most challenging and rewarding experiences of my professional career and it would not be possible without the help of many people.

My deepest gratitude to DK Editorial Team for their guidance and expertise. To Alastair, for believing in me and inviting me on this creative journey, Susan and Amy for their endless dedication behind the scenes, Arran for the beautiful illustrations, and many more.

Thank you to my family for all their love and support, and to my uncle, who taught me to never stop learning. I hope I've made you proud. Thank you to all my friends for rooting for me, René for encouraging me on days that felt the hardest, and Jenny for being the empowering manager and friend she is. Special thanks to Agile Physical Therapy for cheering me on through this process, as well as all my instructors and colleagues who have shaped me as a physical therapist.

Finally, my heartfelt thanks to the readers who have taken the time to delve into the pages of this book to learn and be inspired to move; may it be a worthy addition to your bookshelf.

Publisher acknowledgements

DK would like to thank Alice McKeever for proofreading and Vanessa Bird for indexing.

Picture credits

The publisher would like to thank the following for their kind permission to reproduce their photographs:
(Key: a-above; b-below/bottom; c-centre; f-far; l-left; r-right; t-top)

13 Science Photo Library: Don Fawce (crb). **16 Science Photo Library:** Professors P.M. Motta, P.M. Andrews, K.R. Porter & J. Vial (clb). **25 Science Photo Library:** Biophoto Associates (cla). **35 Science Photo Library:** Thomas Deerinck, Ncmir (cl)

All other images © **Dorling Kindersley**
For further information see: **www.dkimages.com**

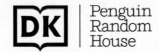

Project Art Editor Amy Child
Project Editor Susan McKeever
Illustrations Arran Lewis

FOR DK
Senior Editor Alastair Laing
Senior Designer Barbara Zuniga
Jacket Coordinator Abi Gain
Senior Production Editor Tony Phipps
Senior Production Controller Luca Bazzoli
Editorial Manager Ruth O'Rourke
Senior Acquistions Editor Becky Alexander
Art Director Maxine Pedliham
Publishing Director Katie Cowan

First published in Great Britain in 2023 by
Dorling Kindersley Limited
DK, One Embassy Gardens, 8 Viaduct Gardens,
London, SW11 7BW

The authorised representative in the EEA is
Dorling Kindersley Verlag GmbH. Arnulfstr. 124,
80636 Munich, Germany

Text copyright © Leada Malek-Salehi 2023
Copyright © 2023 Dorling Kindersley Limited
A Penguin Random House Company
10 9 8 7
017–333491–Nov/2023

A CIP catalogue record for this book
is available from the British Library.
ISBN: 978-0-2415-9340-0

Printed and bound in China

www.dk.com

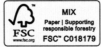

This book was made with Forest
Stewardship Council™ certified
paper – one small step in DK's
commitment to a sustainable future.
**For more information go to
www.dk.com/our-green-pledge**